Nurse Prescribing in Mental Health

DR ADRIAN JONES, RN, BN (HONS), PHD

Nurse Consultant
North Wales NHS Trust & Visiting Reader in
Psychiatric Nursing, Glyndwr University

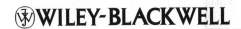

WILEY-BLACKWELL

A John Wiley & Sons, Ltd., Publication

Blackwell Publishing was acquired by John Wiley & Sons in February 2007. Blackwell's publishing programme has been merged with Wiley's global Scientific, Technical, and Medical business to form Wiley-Blackwell.

Registered office
John Wiley & Sons Ltd, The Atrium, Southern Gate, Chichester, West Sussex, PO19 8SQ, United Kingdom

Editorial offices
9600 Garsington Road, Oxford, OX4 2DQ, United Kingdom
2121 State Avenue, Ames, Iowa 50014-8300, USA

For details of our global editorial offices, for customer services and for information about how to apply for permission to reuse the copyright material in this book, please see our website at www.wiley.com/wiley-blackwell.

Library of Congress Cataloging-in-Publication Data
Jones, Adrian, 1969–
Nurse prescribing in mental health / Adrian Jones.
p. ; cm.
Includes bibliographical references and index.
ISBN 978-1-4051-7092-5 (pbk. : alk. paper) 1. Psychiatric nurses—Prescription privileges—Great Britain—Handbooks, manuals, etc. 2. Drug—Prescribing—Great Britian—Handbooks, manuals, etc. I. Title.
[DNLM: 1. Mental Disorders—drug therapy—Great Britain. 2. Mental Disorders—nursing—Great Britain. 3. Nurse's Role—Great Britain. 4. Pharmaceutical Preparations—administration & dosage—Great Britain. 5. Prescriptions, Drug—Great Britain. 6. Psychiatric Nursing—methods—Great Britain. WY 160 J76n 2009]
RC440.J63 2009
616.89′0231—dc22
2008039845

A catalogue record for this book is available from the British Library.

Set in 10/12 Times NRMT by Macmillan Publishing Solutions
Printed in Singapore by Fabulous Printers Pte Ltd

1 2009

Nurse Prescribing in Mental Health

Contents

To my wife Mairead, and my daughter Jessie and son Mikey.

Acknowledgments

Many people have helped to shape this book. Dr Giles Harborne, Consultant Psychiatrist, helped me enormously to become a nurse prescriber, and this support continues in our efforts to improve the patient experience. Dr Rob Poole, Consultant Psychiatrist, provided me with lots of encouragement to write this book and shaped the general direction of travel. Mr Simon Pyke, General Manager, has supported nurse prescribing and remains a strong ally to bring about new ways of working.

There are many friends and colleagues who offered a critique on early chapters, and to name a few, they are Robyn Jones, Tony Scannell, John Carden, Lisa Carden, Julie Mullen, Jaki Bell, John Leung, Debby Land and Rowenna Spencer. My thanks go to them all.

Chapter 1
Mental health nursing:
Our journey and our future

Introduction

This book will begin by looking at the provision of psychiatric care in the past. We need to understand the past to put what we do now into perspective. For some people who read this chapter, it will raise uncomfortable awareness of where nursing has come from. However, our legacy has helped to create the environment for nursing to become an established and respected profession. We draw on many 'drivers for change' that are creating the climate where we now see mental health nurse prescribing and the plethora of services that nurses now lead.

Nurse prescribing is a logical extension of the medical role in response to professional, technological and cultural changes that have occurred over the last 50 years. Nurse prescribing is an innovation for psychiatry; however, the reality is that psychiatric nurses have prescribed medication 'by proxy' for decades, since the introduction of chlorpromazine. Earlier charge nurses would routinely give medication to patients and then have it prescribed at a later time by the doctor. Community nurses alter depot dosage and then have it agreed in team meetings. The point is that although psychiatric nurses have managed, advised and debated medication for decades, they cannot continue this ad hoc procedure as a necessary but only half-acknowledged part of their role. The continued focus on patient safety means that these functions must be legitimised and tied to training and governance structures. Undoubtedly, nurse prescribing will bring about a change for nursing and medical roles, and the benefits will be vast in their impact.

It is argued that medicine and nursing are distinct in their values, training and practices. This has led to tensions and power differences. Nurse prescribing is not some facile attempt to become like doctors. It is rather a challenge for nursing to develop a way of working that meets the needs of patients in settings of their own choice and a new and distinctive way of thinking about the role of drugs in recovery from mental illness.

It is extraordinary that mental health nurses are now embarking on a prescribing career, once the task of the medical superintendent who historically would have been in charge of the hospital staff. The journey through the various stages of psychiatric nursing, from the 'asylum days' right up to the myriad of teams that now make up mental health services, is an interesting one. Professions are changing, and health care too, because of the continuous drive to provide services to more people in different service contexts.

The training of psychiatric professionals has been subject to numerous reviews over the last two decades. This process has helped to extinguish the myth about the supremacy of knowledge and which professional group can lay claim to it. Professional knowledge, and the process of time, which witnesses a relentless march to deprofessionalise it, places a challenge on nursing and medicine. Such a challenge drives nursing forward to take on advanced skills. This book majors on nurse prescribing as one such example although other examples are coming to the fore such as the role of Responsible Clinician under the revised Mental Health Act (DoH 2008b).

A further driver is the role of the patient, or more popularly termed the consumer. Patients have a growing influence over the planning, implementation and evaluation of psychiatric care. People who use mental health services demand greater access, quality and information about the service they receive. Although consumers have often been negative about nurses, they do not distinguish the gap in medical knowledge and intervention to be as wide or necessarily important. We draw out this fact to illustrate a driver for nursing staff that will see them manage and be accountable for even larger aspects of patient care.

The origins of mental health nursing: Asylum attendants

There are institutions that have provided care for people with mental illness for hundreds of years. From 1744 to 1845, care of people with mental illness took place in the workhouse or the private madhouse. The local parish funded this informal form of care. Prior to and up to this period, life was generally organised around the village and so local magistrates and the church managed the care of mental illness. A variety of drivers challenged this arrangement, ranging from scandals in private madhouses to changes in the agricultural and industrial bases of Britain. Efforts were made to put the control and licensing of madhouses under the auspices of the Royal College of Physicians, which was the main medical organisation of the time. This led to medicine being the dominant profession that controlled and regulated people with mental illness.

The 7th Earl of Shaftesbury led the reform of services for lunatics in society and presided over the 1845 Act. In Victorian Britain, there was a massive programme of asylum building. Counties were obliged to establish asylums and admission to them became increasingly regulated through 'commitment' or legal detention. When asylums first opened, they were seen as an exercise in modern humane treatment but very quickly spiralled down into areas of ill treatment (Porter 2002).

The growth of asylums also witnessed an increase in the number of people who were cared for within them. Scull (1979) demonstrated this growth when he examined how many patients per thousand were being detained in 1844 (12.6 per 100000) and then in 1890 (29.2 per 100000). This twofold increase in asylum population was on top of the rising population trend. Quite clearly, the asylums were being used as a method of social disposal.

The development of the asylum model enabled an institutional power base in which the various professions developed an expertise in the treatment of lunatics. Each county asylum was under the control of a physician superintendent, a doctor who had complete administrative and clinical control over the institution. As early as 1841, the Association of Medical Officers of Asylums and Hospitals for the Insane was established, which underwent a series of transformations until it finally became the Royal College of Psychiatrists in 1971.

The day-to-day care of asylum residents was, from the beginning, entrusted to asylum attendants. The working life of asylum attendants was physically demanding with only modest pay and poor working conditions. The attendants were people who were not medically trained and who provided day-to-day care under the supervision of medical superintendents (Brimblecombe 2005). Very soon after the formation of the asylums, there was concern that asylum attendants were generally persons of poor character who provided low-quality care to residents. Medical superintendents tried to improve the way attendants cared for patients by instigating a training scheme and the *Red Handbook* was produced with successive editions printed for the next 60 years. Training of asylum attendants helped to put psychiatric nursing on the starting blocks of becoming a profession. It was not until 1951 that the General Nursing Council took over full responsibility for the training and registration of nurses (Nolan 1998).

Involvement of medical staff in this training also supported the public and professional standing of the medical profession as holding a special body of expertise in the treatment of people with abnormal behaviour. Psychiatric nursing was then seen as the arm of the medical superintendent in this regard.

Thirty years later, in 1982, nurse training curriculum embraced social and psychological theories to help explain mental illness and led to a departure from the medical model. The new curriculum brought the training of psychiatric nurses into line with that of other psychiatric professionals, although this was diluted with the adoption of Project 2000 and its aspirations to increase the professional standing of nursing.

The National Health Service

Until 1948, large mental hospitals were under local authority control. Mental health services became part of the National Health Service (NHS) in 1948, and the slow decline of asylums started immediately. Social welfare policies, coupled with the discovery of new drugs like chlorpromazine, led to an awakening of social psychiatry. It was realised that many of the occupants in hospitals did not need to be there. Changes in society also fuelled the fire for change. The process of 'deinstitutionalisation' led to nursing staff working in an environment where the once-closed wards were opened. Rehabilitation services, day hospitals and outpatient clinics emerged leading to new nursing roles. Coupled with this development was the expectation of using less oppressive practices. Nursing staff needed to embrace a skill set that encompassed therapeutic engagement as opposed to containment.

The development of the NHS created the role of consultant psychiatrists, thus in effect diluting the power of medical superintendents. This was enshrined in law by the 1959 Mental Health Act. The Salmon Report led to the departure from direct supervision by medical superintendents upon the nurses. The reality of the changing relationship did not take place overnight. The concept of multi-disciplinary team working was seen as a driver behind it. The concept of multi-disciplinary team still thrives today where nursing takes place in the myriad of teams providing psychiatric services.

Over the past 30 years, services for adults, substance misuse and older people have been differentiated from the services of an asylum. The onward march towards specialisation started first in the asylums where wards were created for people with alcohol and substance addictions. These wards were seen as separate from the wards for people with mental illness. Nurses and psychiatrists worked in these wards. It was not until the late 1980s that they became completely dislocated from the asylums and developed as stand-alone units or were placed within general hospital grounds. Specialist community services developed in the 1980s. Mental health nurses and psychiatrists were still the main provider for these teams.

The modern crisis in hospital care

The belief in the concept of asylum to manage mental health problems has diminished rapidly. Inpatient care moved from large hospitals to smaller dispersed general hospital units and isolated private facilities. The reality is that the majority of resources continue to be spent on UK hospital care, although the time patients spend in acute psychiatric units is small, some studies pointing towards a mean time of 15 days (Malone *et al.* 2004). There have been relentless attempts to rely less on these units, which continues till date, although we all accept they are an essential component of a modern mental health service.

Mental health nurses are the largest group of staff in hospitals who have 24-h contact with psychiatric patients, and the majority of the professionals still work in many public and private hospitals and residential homes in the UK. What is disappointing are the countless studies even today demonstrating that nurses are reluctant to engage with adult and older people or provide therapeutic activities for them (Standing Nursing and Midwifery Advisory Committee 1999; Sainsbury Centre for Mental Health 2003, 2005).

The care vacuum that has developed on psychiatric wards today is a symptom of the malaise that had developed within psychiatry in general. Problems like understaffing and rising acuity increased detention rates. Dual diagnosis – to name but a few – exerted a fundamental need to review just what inpatient care should look like (Healthcare Commission 2007a; Royal College of Psychiatrists 2007).

It seems difficult to imagine that psychiatric nurses would be able to manage patient care episodes on top of the added responsibilities that come with assessment and treatment encompassed within nurse prescribing. However, this must be seen within the context of acute wards staying in their present state. Acute wards are changing and the fluidity of the system requires health professionals to be more accessible than ever before. Psychiatrists visiting wards once a week is becoming difficult to sustain given the rising acuity and necessity for quicker decision making for home treatment. Care arrangements will be increasingly made across the spectrum of health care for nursing staff to admit, diagnose, treat and discharge from hospitals. Nurse prescribing will help to oil the wheels of change and give nurses the tools to carry out these new tasks. Radical change is still required within our acute inpatient units to make them fit for purpose, but the future is certainly promising for nurses who work in hospital settings.

Care in the community

The process of deinstitutionalisation witnessed one of the biggest social advancements in the management of patients. The closure of wards in hospitals shifted the base where nurses and psychiatrists worked and began to change the relationship between nurses and psychiatrists (Brimblecombe 2005). In essence, as patients were discharged from hospitals and the concept of care moved from containment to therapeutic engagement, the location of nursing also shifted to community services. Hence, from the 1980s, there were a rapid expansion of community services and differentiated services to meet particular needs. Nurses increased their levels of autonomy over the management of patient care.

The most visible consequence of community care has been the establishment of community mental health teams. They were first established in the 1960s and gained prominence in the 1990s. When a community mental health team works well, it is able to harness the skills of many team members and disciplines to assess and deliver care. Overall, the dominance of the medical model in decision making and direction over care has been complemented by the influence of social work and nursing perspectives. One could argue that the movement of care from the hospital setting to a person's home led to a period of professional uncertainty for nursing staff too, as they competed with social work for position within the expanding community team.

The primary reason for establishing a community mental health team was to deliver more cost-effective approaches to care. However, early teams were found to be ineffective in managing staff resources towards caring for patients with a serious mental illness (Onyett *et al.* 1994). Even today, the evidence base for community mental health teams is inadequate and reveals no great difference in the reduction of suicides compared to non-team standard care (Malone *et al.* 2007).

In the mid-1990s, there were a number of high-profile cases where people with mental illness went on to kill members of the public, one notable example being Christopher Clunis (Ritchie *et al.* 1994). This added to the perception that community-based services had failed. However, the community mental health team did enable nursing staff to receive referrals from general practitioners. This had the effect of increasing the professional stature of community nurses but consequently raised concerns within the medical profession, as their spheres of influence became challenged.

Growing resentment with the ineffective community mental health team led to the government producing a national service framework and advocating other types of teams to develop, such as assertive community treatment and crisis resolution home treatment teams (DoH 1999; DoH/CSIP 2007). At the front end of service provision, nursing staff are the clinicians who will deal with crisis situations. Nurses working in adult and older persons' services increasingly prioritise, formulate and treat without the patient ever being seen by the psychiatrist. The old assumption that doctors should be involved with all major decisions has collapsed. It is also fair to say that the expansion of community-based services has helped to bolt down a less reliant service response on hospital beds (Fawcett & Karban 2005).

The movement of care from the traditional asylum base also saw the emergence of independent sectors in providing care for people requiring differing levels of security; interestingly, these sectors have occupied the market in proving costly continuing care. Unlike the state facilities they have replaced, these private institutions are predominantly led by nurses but staffed by nursing assistants.

The movement of care into a community-based setting placed nursing staff into an arena where they had to work alongside other statutory and voluntary sector agencies. This in itself has led to both positive and negative consequences not only for the care and treatment of patients but also for the profession of nursing. However, the reality of health care over the last few decades has been a splintering of the care episode; nursing has tried to exploit areas where it can take on ever-larger elements of that care. In other words, the destiny of mental health nursing has grown from a reliance and dominance with medicine but is now shaped by costs and service user needs.

Chronic diseases and the overall burden of health

The most common form of disability is mental health problems. Up to 27% of Europeans experience mental illness in any given year (Wittchen & Jacobi 2005). Projections indicate that by 2020, depression will be the highest ranked disease in the developed world (World Health Organization 2001). Mental health nurses make up the largest proportion of the workforce in the UK, which places them in an ideal position to improve the care for people who are in need for services.

Chronic disease management describes a system that prioritises care for a group of patients who are high users of care and who are then specifically 'case managed' through the whole system of care (Katon *et al.* 2001; Gask 2005). The whole system speaks in terms of primary and secondary care but would prefer to see it as a complete unbroken care pathway (Wanless 2002). The second strand to chronic disease management is the role of the consumer. Policy has been put forward that creates roles for nursing staff, such as 'community matrons', to empower patients to take decisions regarding their care and treatment (DoH 2005a). The concept of 'direct payments' where people can decide how to buy their own community support furthers this point (CSIP-NIMHE 2006).

Crucially, the concept of disease management sees the disease split up into a triangle approach. At the top of the triangle are the most complex patients who have an uncertain diagnosis and pathological pathway and thus require expert management from consultant medical staff (Katon *et al.* 2001). It is reasonable to argue that 75% of the diagnostic group can be managed to varying degrees by nursing staff. Although the aim of disease management is to provide better management of patient care, it has led to a direct driver for nursing staff to develop and further extend their skills into the domain of medical staff.

Another policy driver is the concept of nurse-led discharge where suitably trained nurses follow patient progress and execute discharge when the patients reach discharge markers identified in their care pathway (DoH 2004a). Teams or individuals, like home treatment teams, discharge nurse posts, and nurse practitioners have been trained to carry out these types of functions. Again this departs from the era where medical staff took decisions about admission and discharge of patients. For example, the situation still arises today where psychiatrists discharge patients on a certain day of the week, not unsurprisingly falling on the 'ward round' day.

A major challenge with the chronic disease model is for nursing and medical staff to depart from a generalist position and take on a specialist position (Gask 2005). When nursing takes on specialised functions like admission, treatment and discharge from parts of the care pathway, it ultimately leads to changes in the way medical staff work. The key difference with this model is that the nurse delivers care that cuts across the boundaries between hospital and community services. This means that for some patients, you are just as likely to find nurses managing patient care in a hospital setting than in a community setting. Changes to the law enabling nurses to prescribe medication really makes this way of thinking possible, which will be further catalysed by changes to the revised Mental Health Act. The next service innovation for mental health nurses will be the role of a responsible clinician (DoH 2008b). The role of a responsible clinician, coupled with being an independent prescriber, will allow some nurses to be employed to deliver complete packages of care. This will be truly the profession coming of age and will be able to support the longer term management of the disease burden facing the UK.

Role of the consumer

Over the past two decades, the NHS has gone through a sea change towards a consumerist ethos within health care. A business management agenda has attempted to challenge the foundations of healthcare provision by empowering the user of care (Griffiths 1988). The Patient's Charter was an example of putting the rights of consumers in health care in the centre of care provision (DoH 1996). Recovery, which resonates strongly in mental health, has been a further development where recipients of health care have reacted against a system that for too long has traded on maintenance (Turner 2002). The DoH (1999c, 2001) has politicised this mindset where services are now supposed to be recovery focused. Patients can now receive direct payments so that they can have choice and purchase their own care packages (CSIP-NIMHE 2006). This business, consumer-driven agenda will be pushed further with the emergence of foundation NHS trusts.

But has consumer participation made any real difference? Consumer satisfaction has gained widespread recognition and, increasingly, is being seen as a driver to shape service delivery (Rose 2001). The challenge is to overcome the tokenistic impression of consumer involvement in all aspects of mental health care (Lammers & Happell 2004). A key battleground is who actually owns the patient record. It seems paradoxical that in today's climate of patient self-management, clinicians are reticent about handing control over to patients to write in their own notes or to see and comment about what clinicians are saying about them in the clinical record (Happell *et al.* 2002).

Early debates have centred on the validity of collecting views from patients on their experiences of care (Fitzpatrick 1991). However, the credibility of this claim has been dismantled as clear evidence has emerged that people with mental health problems can exercise and articulate their opinion on their experiences of health care (Noble *et al.* 2001). Patients will increasingly be concerned with exercising choice over the provider of their care, with less attention paid to profession and more to the quality of the service and time spent with the clinician. A systematic review of the views of mental health patients on receiving care from professional staff found that patients wanted staff to use a range of interventions to positively influence their mental health. This was irrespective of profession as long as the clinician concerned was trained appropriately and was competent to deliver the intervention (Noble *et al.* 2001).

Patients would like to spend more time with nursing staff, discussing their diagnosis and treatment options. Patients want nurses to be both professional and ordinary in their approach (Barker *et al.* 1999). This may explain why early nurse-prescribing research indicates that patients prefer the prescribing advice from nurses to that from doctors because of the different social language used (Luker *et al.* 1998).

One of the main benefits through empowerment of the user has been more information being given to the patient during the clinical encounter (Baker 1998). However, it is questionable if this can be said for people with mental illness, who have been perceived as being disempowered within society (Brandon 1991). Godfrey (1996) found that psychiatric patients were not perceived as active partners in the care planning process. However, this has also been noted in other settings such as primary care. For McIver (1999), there was a perception that users had trouble in being an active participant and were not particularly committed towards changing service provision. Behind the drive for consumer power, there is an underlying assumption that patients want to be involved in decision making, although this is not always the case. In many respects, the rhetoric of consumerism seems to be overshadowed by the complexity of the relationship that patients assume and want when they are the recipients of health care.

The rise in consumerism appears to have greater impact on those who provide the services. Quite frankly, some clinicians feel threatened by a more interactive user. Lupton (1997) observed this in a study of the relationship between general practitioners and patients. Respondents spoke about a sense of the profession being 'devalued' and being held as more accountable to the needs of the patient. This is a positive feature of the rise in consumerism and challenges the perception of 'they must know what they are doing' attitude, which features in the clinical encounter (Baker 1998). A similar trend was observed between general practitioners and people who were depressed, with the low levels of involvement the latter felt in the consultation regarding their treatment options (Loh *et al.* 2006). Similarly, educators of mental health nurses were equally uncomfortable conceding ground as to who were the real experts in mental health care (Felton & Stickley 2004). Other studies on mental health nurses also demonstrated that patients are involved in selecting the right type of medication and deciding whether they should comply with treatment (McCann *et al.* 2008). A key factor may be the absence of skills in clinicians to involve patients in care-related decisions (Gravel *et al.* 2006). This is the key challenge for nurse prescribers as they enter the new world of patient-driven services.

There have been studies on what patients think about their inpatient care experience. Rogers & Pilgrim (1994) reported that over half of patients were either satisfied or very satisfied with their inpatient nursing care. Interestingly, 32% of patients ranked the helpfulness of nurses higher than that of psychiatrists. Again, what is being drawn out here is that patients are beginning to distinguish their preferences for a professional group. This is in contrast to a widely held view that patients would naturally prefer to have aspects of their care from doctors.

Patients are being encouraged to be active players in what medication they take. The key point here is that people are moving from being a passive recipient of care to being an active participant (Happell *et al.* 2002). A recent DoH (2008a) initiative on medication management identifies very clearly the responsibility mental health nurses have in empowering patients to question the steps in medication management. Patients are urged to ask questions about the role of medication, its safety profile, how the medication should be taken, side effects, information leaflets, how to stop taking it and the alternatives to medication. Patients armed with these questions will present a big challenge to nurses who may not have the knowledge or interpersonal awareness to engage in such a debate. However, patients want, expect and deserve this kind of interaction, given it is them who are taking the medication.

Conclusion

The historical journey for mental health nurses began in the asylums where they were under the control of medical staff. The history of psychiatric nursing is important, as it gives the context to why nurses behave in the way they do in light of new advancements such as nurse prescribing.

The number of mental health nurses has grown since 1997 with investment in nurse training opportunities and employment prospects upon qualification (DoH 2000). Patients value the role that nurses play in promoting their recovery. It is significant that in the latest consultation exercise for mental health nursing, the most frequently identified role that would benefit patients was nurse prescribing (DoH 2006c). The development of nurse consultant and specialist practitioner posts will drive forward the future roles and professional footprint of mental health nursing as they take on more substantive aspects of mental health work.

Transfer of care and treatment in to community settings highlighted the importance of teamwork. Teamwork can lead to problems with professional identity, conflict between the professions and defensive practice. However, this should be seen as an opportunity for change. Training and development may lead to clinicians adapting to the market requirement to meet the needs of patients by delivering interventions that do not fit the traditional professional roles.

This chapter has drawn out the history of mental health nursing. Nursing is seen as a relationship between nurses and patients. Patients expect this relationship and are disappointed when they are deprived of it in the healthcare setting. Patients want nurses to listen, empathise and generally support them with regard to their mental health problems, and offer harsh criticism when this does not happen.

Economics is also driving healthcare provision and hence the growth in disease management. Consumer demand is changing the way patients want to be treated and by whom. Nurse prescribing is not just about advancing the professional agenda of nursing. It is about meeting economic and consumer demands. Patients will be less concerned about professional grandstanding and will take the road of pragmatism. Mental health nurses, as they have demonstrated in the past, will have to grasp the new clothes that are being laid before them. Nurse prescribing is certainly a key activity for future clinicians.

A further question raised in this chapter is whether nurses will want to take on these new skills. The number of mental health nurses who are being trained to use prescriptive authority is growing; there is emerging evidence of new ways of working that meet the needs of patients. The green shoots of innovation need support and encouragement and this starts with valuing the present and future roles that nurses can offer the clinical encounter.

Chapter 2
Mental health nurse prescribing:
The UK and the World

Introduction

Nurses have prescriptive authority in a number of countries across the globe. Legislative changes in different countries led to varied adaptation of the nurse-prescribing role. The UK was a relatively new entrant into this field of practice and has developed different types of nurse prescriber. Drivers for nurse prescribing in the UK include quicker access to health care and more informed patients about their treatments. Many policy directions and mental health reviews have been published to support this new way of working. This chapter also reviews a patient group direction. Patient group directions are not a form of prescribing; they are an added administrative form of giving medication and are underutilised in mental health services.

What factors have led to nurse prescribing?

The answer to this question deserves some discussion before the detail of the legislation is reviewed. The UK government have stated unequivocally that the aim of nurse prescribing is to maximise access and choice to patients who use health services by increasing the flexibility of the skills of the workforce (DoH 1989, 2000, 2003, 2006b). This assertion has been supported by a number of research studies (Jones 2007a,b; Nolan & Bradley 2007; Stenner & Courtenay 2008). The principles that have underpinned the decision to extend nurse prescribing have been the following.

- Improve patient safety
- Provide greater access and choice
- Add flexibility into healthcare provision
- Deliver better medicines management
- Extend and not replace multidisciplinary care

Nurse–patient relationship

Mental health nursing focuses on the importance of the relationship for the assessment and treatment of the patient. One of the greatest strengths of this profession is the increased access to the patient and the family members. This enables the nurse to detect changes in mental state and add to overall case management responsibilities whether in hospital or in the community. This is why nurse prescribing offers such promise in terms of patient monitoring and treatment. The nurse prescriber is able to combine the social world of the patient with the medical requirement for treatment. A survey of mental health nurses specifically identified the prospect of greater choice for the patient as a result of nurse prescribing (Nolan & Bradley 2007).

Nurse prescribing bringing about new ways of working

Very early on, nurse prescribing has been seen as a political manoeuvre to bring about new ways of working, with the stated intentions to provide benefits to patients in terms of choice and access to medication (Jones & Jones 2005, 2006). Changes to the way nurses and doctors work, primarily influenced by the increased specialisation of doctors, have been an important factor in the UK. The UK government (DoH 1999b) advocated in the report 'Making a difference' that nurse prescribing should be seen as part of the modernising agenda for the nursing profession, and further recommended that over half of all registered nurses in England should have varying degrees of prescriptive authority (DoH 2000).

The commitment to equip psychiatric nurses with supplementary and independent prescribing responsibilities heralds an opportunity to significantly increase the capacity of the workforce across the whole spectrum of mental health services. Incumbent within this is an extension to the skill set and an enablement of nurses to take a greater lead in the reform of health care.

When we talk about nurse prescribing, we also reflect on new ways of working. New ways of working is where responsibility for delivering interventions is distributed amongst the team (DoH 2007a,b). This then enables those workers who are the most highly trained, skilled and paid spend their time looking after the most complicated people. This is a commendable outcome and helps to usher in an era where psychiatrists can begin to supervise nursing colleagues to deliver packages of care for patients. It must be remembered that unidiscipline supervision has been the norm for mental health nursing. It seems likely that nurse prescribing has helped to put flesh on the bones for new ways of working.

Working differently does place a challenge on both psychiatrists and mental health nurses. For some nurses, it may uncover a lack of confidence to take on roles traditionally undertaken by medical staff. Lack of confidence comes from inadequate training opportunities (e.g. being physical health assessments), lack of supervision and mentoring and a perception of organisational ignorance towards acceptable risk taking. All take their toll on how nurses approach their work.

There have been a number of drivers that have led to nurses being granted prescriptive authority. Workforce changes, most notably that of junior doctors, and the requirements of the European Working Time Directive have placed challenges on services. Modernising nursing careers is also a driver to make sure that nurses take their rightful place in managing episodes of care and the flow of patient care (DoH 2006e). Hospital at Night is one such high-profile initiative. Hospital at Night is the term adopted nationally for looking at redesigning services, introducing new rules and extended practice to address the impact of reducing doctor's hours.

Better medicines management

Will nurse prescribing lead to improved prescribing decisions? Medication is a high-risk area. An alarming number of 55 deaths per year and 392 deaths per year have been associated with antipsychotic and antidepressant drugs, respectively (NPSA 2006). Risks may well be because of system errors or lack of adherence to best practice, either produced locally or nationally. It is too early to tell whether nurse prescribing would lead to less prescriptive errors noted in the NPSA (2006) report, although, by tradition, nurses are more likely to follow guidelines and stay within their competency framework.

A report carried out by the Healthcare Commission (2007b) points out that mental health patients are routinely prescribed high doses of antipsychotic medication, subjected to medication regimes with polypharmacy and with little attention to physical health and side-effect monitoring. The report puts this down to poor monitoring of the effects of medication and the need to rationalise medication when crisis points are over or titration has taken place. The review demonstrated that national guidelines for the management of major conditions and for prescribing medications were not followed consistently. Given that psychiatrists are the main prescribing body when patients are in hospital, the report suggests much more rigorous control over the quality of the prescribing intervention.

The Healthcare Commission (2007b) report also looked at the area of mental health nurse prescribing. Of the 35 trusts that took part in the review, 26 had nurse prescribers totalling 187, and of these 187 nurse prescribers, 81 reported that they prescribed 'at least once per week'. Concern raised by the report was that nurse prescribers must maintain their competence by being in situations where they routinely prescribe medication in appropriate situations.

A matter of concern is that only 52% of trusts reported a procedure for checking competency to prescribe. The report recommended that trusts maximised the benefits that may accrue from supplementary and independent prescribing, and was in many respects helpful for the nurse-prescribing journey. The challenge will be when nurse-prescribing decisions are considered alongside medical prescribing decisions and if the outcomes described above are any different.

Nurse prescribing enables the opportunity for nurses to educate patients about their medication. Imparting information is a skilful activity. The higher amount of time in contact with the patient may enable better opportunities to negotiate treatment plans and therefore concordance with treatment. Arguably, the framework of supplementary prescribing may lead to medicines being delivered far safer given the level of discussion that is required. The process of medicines management becomes explicit within the prescribing process. The higher amounts of contact between the patient and the nurse prescriber may lead to quicker decisions about medication. This may save time for patients.

Nurse prescribing across the world

The descriptor term *nurse prescribing* is correct but the actual activity is different and set by the needs of the country (ICN 2004). Nurse prescribing in its most liberal sense has been adopted in developing countries (Miles *et al.* 2006). A brief overview of various countries that have adopted nurse prescribing will help to give the reader an understanding of its application in the UK.

The USA

In the USA, nurse prescribing has been part of the health system since the 1960s. It was of help in those areas where specialist doctors and nurses choose not to work (Bailey 1999). Each state differs in the boundaries of practice (Kaas & Markley 1998). In 27 states, nurses can determine the scope of practice with no supervisory relationship with a psychiatrist. In 14 states, a nurse requires a collaborative agreement with a psychiatrist, and in 5 states the scope of practice is supervised by doctors (Phillips 2005).

The context of the prescribing relationship is different in the USA because citizens can choose the provider of treatment. Systems of insurance also reimburse the provider of care and, in effect, because nursing reimbursement is cheaper than that of doctors, insurers are supportive of nurse prescribers.

The training to become a nurse prescriber is governed by each state. An example is of nurses in the state of Colorado who first undertake a masters degree and then require 1800 h of medical supervision from a psychiatrist. Once qualified, the nurse practitioner works in a collaborative model. The model sets out the types of patients that can be seen by the nurse practitioner (Jones 2006e).

Canada

In Canada, nurse prescribing started in the 1990s. Similar to the USA, there is no uniform parameter for prescriptive authority. The origin of nurse prescribing was in primary care and in isolated geographical areas, largely because of the absence of medical staff perpetuated by increasing specialisation. Nurse prescribers are regulated by the provincial areas and this sets forth activities such as making a diagnosis and prescribing treatment that are deemed to be 'controlled acts'. When nurses complete the required training, they become 'primary care practitioners'; this registration allows them to diagnose and treat across the health spectrum for patients and families.

Nurse prescribing in Ontario lays out the limits of prescriptive practice and the type of consultation relationship nurse prescribers have with doctors. A definition of the level of the intervention required from a doctor includes an opinion, a recommendation, a concurrent intervention or the immediate transfer of care. Doctors assure the organisation or the provincial area of nursing competency (College of Nurses of Ontario 2005a,b).

New Zealand

In New Zealand, nurse prescribing started in 1999 as a result of the nursing profession taking on advanced roles (Lim *et al.* 2007). Similar to other countries, careful consideration of the safety and professional issues was made by the health department (New Zealand Ministry of Health 1997). Care of the elderly was one of the first areas to help improve access to health care in rural areas (New Zealand Ministry of Health 1998). In New Zealand, preparation for nurses to become a nurse prescriber includes 5 years of experience in a specialist area and a masters degree.

Australia

Australia has developed nurse prescribing through nurse practitioner posts, particularly psychiatric liaison services and nurse-led clinics (Wand & White 2007). A number of prescribing models have been developed. An example of nurse prescribing can be seen in Western Australia and New South Wales where the nurse works within a collaborative model of practice. The nurse prescribes medication by following a protocol. An example of this model is seen in Victoria where nurses are authorised to prescribe medication for emergency care situations via a protocol in rural settings. In other states of Australia, nurses are permitted to initiate medication, and this is controlled to specifying the medication and the dose (National Nursing and Nursing Education Taskforce 2006a,b). This form of prescribing appears similar to patient group directives in the UK.

Sweden

In Sweden, only district nurses can prescribe medication and this has been in place since 1994. The main reason for its introduction was to lessen the demand on overstretched general practitioner services. The medical profession was initially concerned that more medication would be prescribed by these nurses (Nilsson 1994). District nurses have experienced an increased sense of job satisfaction in being a nurse prescriber (Wilhelmsson & Foldevi 2003). There is no prescribing activity for mental health conditions.

Ireland

Nurses in Ireland have started to prescribe medication in 2007. Although support was indicated for nurses to prescribe, only 14% of nurses who responded to a survey supported independent prescribing (An Bord Altranais 2005). For clinical nurse specialists, concerns about litigation underpin reluctance to implement the approach (Lockwood & Fealy 2008). Wells *et al.* (*In press*) found that community psychiatric nurses were 'ambivalent' about the value of extending nurse prescribing to a community setting. The reason for introducing nurse prescribing was to improve productivity in the health system and promote greater access to health care. In Ireland, nurses prescribe medication by following collaborative practice agreements. This is very similar to a clinical management plan. The collaborative practice agreement is between the nurse prescriber, the doctor and the employing organisation. It sets out the clinical experience of the nurse prescriber, their scope of competency and a defined area where the nurse can prescribe, including the diagnosis of the patient and the types of medicines permissible to be prescribed (An Bord Altranais 2005). In some ways, this advances the prescribing model for the UK in that it sets out the types of patients to be overseen by the nurse prescriber.

Holland

In Holland, mental health nurses have started to be trained as nurse prescribers since 2007. They are masters prepared nurses and have authority to prescribe within their area of practice. The Dutch method has been to wrap nurse prescribing within a nurse practitioner model of care. The Dutch Parliament has accepted the specialist nurse-prescribing proposal; however, this still requires the law to be changed. In the meantime, nurses are also able to prescribe medication for drugs such as lithium for mood stabilisation. The nurses do not need to undergo a specialist training programme, although they are required to undergo supervision of a psychiatrist.

Botswana, Uganda and South Africa

The situation in Africa is very different to the Western progression of nurse prescribing. Nurses are often the primary and only care giver in low-income countries and take on roles like prescribing to deliver the treatment people need to stay alive. Examples such as prescribing for human immunodeficiency virus (HIV) and AIDS in hospice settings capture the true extent of exclusion from services in countries like Uganda (Jagwe & Merriman 2007; Jack & Merriman 2008). Nurses may not have any training and would lack a legislative framework. Nurses would work in rural settings where medical supervision may be limited or not available (Miles *et al.* 2006).

In some African countries such as Botswana, the idea of nurses prescribing treatment for curable diseases was accepted into the fabric of health care (Ngcongco & Stark 1986). As time progressed, nurses were trained to deliver nurse prescribing alongside wider public health interventions. In South Africa, a licence is granted to nurse prescribers by the Pharmacy Council of South Africa following a period of competency-based training (Miles *et al.* 2006). A controlled trial showed that the practice of prescribing is better in trained nurses compared to nurses that had not received any training (Meyer *et al.* 2001). For under-resourced countries, this not only is a huge step forward for the population but also shows how nurses can be at the forefront of this public health agenda.

Global expansion

Without doubt, nurse prescribing is a global development for nursing. Each country has progressed nurse prescribing because of unmet service need. There are not only commonalities in the form of prescriptive authority but also differences in training, legislation and acceptance. A major driver for nurse prescribing is the rural dimension of health care where people live in underserved areas and have needs that are not met. Nurse prescribing has flourished in these areas and the model of prescribing becomes ever less regulated.

For countries that have poor resources and limited doctors, the need for nurses that can prescribe presents an ethical dilemma. Many people would not be able to receive curable treatment if nurses do not give them the medication. African nations have however developed the legislative frameworks to train nurses to prescribe medication. This is where the World Health Organisation and the International Council of Nurses can help to present broad regulatory agreement so that nurse prescribing adds value to health outcomes and does less harm to the communities they serve (Miles *et al.* 2006).

In the UK, the Nursing & Midwifery Council maintains a record of all registered nurses and those annotated as an independent or supplementary prescriber. There are approximately 50,000 mental health nurses with about 650 registered as a nurse prescriber. The number of nurse prescribers is growing annually, fully supported by policy and service demand.

Nurse prescribing in the UK

Before 1990, only doctors and dentists were able to prescribe prescription-only medicines. The origin of nurse prescribing in the UK can be traced back to Baroness Julia Cumberlege's review of 'community nursing' in 'Neighbourhood nursing: A focus for care' (Department of Health and Social Security 1986). It was found that district nurses were competent in their knowledge of certain procedures requiring bandages. Prescribing of bandages did not require the specialist knowledge of a doctor. This led to the founding of an advisory board led by Dr June Crown to explore the implications of nurse prescribing and the recommendations from this report were called the first Crown Report (DoH 1989). Hence, the concept of nurse prescribing was born where nurses could prescribe independently medical treatments from a limited list and for a defined group of patients. Legislation enabling nurses to prescribe medication in this way was contained within the Medicinal Products: Prescribing by Nurses etc. Act 1992.

The then government asked Dr June Crown to reconsider the prescribing of medication by nurses. She prepared another report that was called the second Crown Report, which was published in 1999 (DoH 1999b).

This led the way for a more extended form of prescribing, later to be named supplementary prescribing, which was intended for nurses and pharmacists to work with doctors in the management of chronic diseases. This report recommended that prescribing should be extended to new professional groups. The report also introduced the concept of an independent prescriber.

It is important to note slight differences between the pace of change for nurse prescribing within England and Wales. The primary legislation for medicines management applies across the UK. Slight differences in pace can be accounted for because secondary legislation was required in Wales for nurse prescribing to be adopted. Unlike England, Wales did not accept the type of prescriber called an extended independent nurse prescriber. At the time of writing, both England and Wales have adopted supplementary and independent prescribing roles in a range of mental health services and settings.

Types of nurse prescriber

Many changes to legislation, training and scope of prescribing have led to four main types of nurse prescribers, different training routes accounting for different parameters of prescribing activity (see Table 2.1).

Nurse prescribing from the extended formulary

The extended formulary has arisen and developed over the years with more and more drugs and conditions being specified. It was originally designed for practice nurses and district nurses. On first sight one would not consider the formulary terribly useful for mental health settings. However, if one were to take that view, you would lose sight of the potential benefits of mental health nurses being able to treat more aspects of the patient's condition and so take on a holistic approach to mental health care. More often than not medical conditions listed in the extended formulary coexist in mental health settings, particularly older persons and learning disability units and services. Examples relevant for practice include medication for constipation.

Table 2.1 Types of nurse-prescribing qualification course

V100	Nurses with V100 qualification were previously known as health visitor and district nurses who prescribed from the formulary. They are now known as a community practitioner with a specialist qualification.
V200	Nurses with V200 qualification were previously known as nurses who had extended formulary-prescribing rights. They are now known as supplementary prescribers.
V300	Nurses with V300 qualification were previously known as nurses who could be an extended formulary prescriber, supplementary prescriber and independent prescriber.
V150	Nurses with V150 qualification work as a community practitioner nurse prescriber and can prescribe from the community practitioner formulary.

Mental health nurses who have completed the V300 independent or supplementary prescribing course are also able to prescribe from the extended formulary provided they are competent to treat the condition listed and that the governance arrangements have been agreed that allow the nurse prescriber to use the drug listed in the formulary for use in the setting. An example would be of an independent prescriber prescribing chlordiazepoxide for patients diagnosed with acute signs of alcohol dependence syndrome [chlordiazepoxide is licensed for the treatment of alcohol withdrawal (BNF 2008)].

Community practitioner formulary

Advances to the type of prescriber have been put in place. A training programme is proposed that would prepare registered nurses who did not have a specialist practitioner qualification to prescribe from a community practitioner formulary. Plans are in place for nurses who have undertaken this shortened period of training to then carry forward the training for supplementary and independent prescribing qualifications. The benefits for nurses to undertake this programme of study is that they will be able to use their skills in prescribing a limited range of drugs as part of their prescribing career. Nurse prescribing is a competency-based activity that needs to be continually assessed with extension to prescriptive authority as competency develops.

Supplementary prescribing

Supplementary prescribing first started in England in 2003 (DoH 2003; National Prescribing Centre 2005a), and a year later in Wales. The agreed-upon definition for supplementary prescribing: 'a voluntary prescribing partnership between the independent prescriber (doctor) and supplementary prescriber (nurse) to implement an agreed specific clinical management plan with the patient's agreement' (DoH 2006a). In order for a clinical management plan to be valid, the patient and psychiatrist must agree for a nurse to prescribe medicines; the psychiatrist must have assessed the patient; and a treatment plan must be agreed (Table 2.2).

Supplementary prescribing is defined as a partnership between the independent prescriber, who is a doctor, and the supplementary prescriber, who is either a nurse or a pharmacist, to implement an agreed patient-specific clinical management plan. It must be remembered that supplementary prescribing was intended for use in the management of chronic conditions (DoH 2003). On a superficial level, this would exclude hospital-based presentations, as conditions by their nature of presentation are likely to be acute. However, the parameters of supplementary prescribing also include acute episodes that occur as part of the chronic condition. Medicines that can be prescribed within a clinical management plan are fairly broad ranging, hence the flexibility of this form of prescribing (Table 2.3).

Table 2.2   Components for a clinical management plan

Demographics	Name of the patient, signed by all three parties with the beginning date.
Disease	Illness to be treated, range of medications to be used, citation of evidence-based guidelines.
Drugs	Sensitivities, coexisting medication conditions, contraindications, potential adverse drug reactions.
Limitations	Reasons why the clinical management plan would end and what to do in the event.
Consent	Supplementary prescribing is a consensual agreement between all parties.

Table 2.3   Types of drugs that can be prescribed by a supplementary prescriber

General sales list	This includes pharmacy medicines, devices, foods and appliances.
Prescription-only medication	This includes controlled drugs except Schedule I drugs.
Off-label prescribing	Licensed medication for unlicensed use.
Black triangle drugs	A newly licensed drug where all adverse drug reactions need to be reported.

Medications that the supplementary prescriber is unable to prescribe are as follows.

- Medicines that are restricted by the General Medical Services Regulations – Schedule 10 and 11
- Unlicensed drugs, unless they are part of a clinical trial with a certificate or exemption
- Drugs subject to the Misuse of Drugs Regulations Act

Supplementary prescribing is a useful prescribing framework for chronic diseases such as schizophrenia and bipolar disorder (Jones & Jones 2007a,b, 2008b). Mental health conditions also occur with complex pathologies such as diabetes and cardiovascular disease. Some nurses may feel uncomfortable to prescribe for the full range of conditions that the patients present with, which is an understandable and defensible position.

The doctor has a range of responsibilities within this supplementary prescribing relationship and it includes the initial diagnostic formulation of the patient. The doctor will also agree to the range of medication that can be used by the supplementary prescriber and an undertaking to support the supplementary prescribing nurse to carry out this prescribing function.

The implementation of supplementary prescribing is most suited for:

(1) treatment of long-term conditions where reviews can be carried out between consultations with the doctor;

(2)   close working relationships required between the supplementary prescriber and the medical practitioner.

Supplementary prescribing was to be different from the extended formulary independent prescribing as there were no legal restrictions on the types of conditions the supplementary prescriber could prescribe for. The whole idea is for the clinical management plan to be as simple as possible but the administrative requirements sometimes preclude this. Either the nurse or the doctor can write the clinical management plan, although a discussion should take place between all three parties following diagnosis. These steps can delay the process. Clinical management plans should be reviewed on an annual basis or earlier if the condition warrants.

Completing the clinical management plan

The clinical management plan is the cornerstone of supplementary prescribing. It sets out an agreement between the nurse, patient and the psychiatrist. The clinical management plan has a number of categories to be completed when all three parties agree to the process (see Table 2.3). The clinical management plan is signed and filed in the patient's notes. It is good practice to attach the clinical management plan to the drug chart for ease of access. If the patient is being managed in primary care, a copy of the clinical management plan should be sent to the patient's general practitioner.

There is a section on the clinical management plan that allows the prescriber to identify the guidelines that are being referred to. Major diagnostic conditions such as dementia, depression and bipolar disorder have specific National Institute for Clinical Excellence (NICE) guidelines. The prescriber may also be governed by trust medication protocols, which spell out how drugs should be prescribed. These should be noted on the clinical management plan.

Independent nurse prescribing

Prescriptive authority was extended in the UK for three main reasons: to increase access to medicinal products, to increase patient choice and to make better use of healthcare resources (DoH 2006a). Independent prescribing can be defined as 'prescribing by a practitioner (e.g. doctor, dentist, nurse, pharmacist) responsible and accountable for the assessment of patients with undiagnosed or diagnosed conditions and for decisions about the clinical management required, including prescribing' (DoH 2006b). The government did consult on extending the formulary, and without surprise, the medical profession was sceptical in some quarters and hostile in others. However, that said the Medicines for Human Use (Prescribing) (Miscellaneous Amendments) Order of May 2006 was passed, enabling nurses who had passed the nurse-prescribing course to prescribe any licensed medication for any medical condition within their scope of competence.

The scope of medication that can be prescribed is far-reaching. Independent prescribers are able to prescribe controlled drugs but only for defined medical conditions. An example is the prescription of chlordiazepoxide hydrochloride for alcohol withdrawal symptoms. Interestingly, lorazepam, a drug commonly prescribed to control arousal in psychosis, is not permitted to be prescribed by an independent prescriber. In fact, independent prescribers are not allowed to prescribe medications that have not been licensed in the UK. They can prescribe drugs off-label so long as they inform the patient about this practice and the nurse can defend this prescription against standard practice.

All nurses who completed the nurse-prescribing course in England were eligible to practice as an independent prescriber. Slight differences in Wales were proposed where all nurses trained on the course before October 2006 had to undergo a further period of training. Nurses trained outside the principality of Wales also have to pass a numeracy exam before they can practice in the Welsh Trust.

The implementation of independent prescribing is different to supplementary prescribing in that:

(1) prescribing is within the competency of the nurse to diagnose and treat certain conditions;
(2) the independent prescriber works remotely from the doctor.

The key difference with independent prescribing is that the nurse holds a greater level of autonomy, although this does not mean that the nurse is left to manage all aspects of the patient's condition. Doctors may have previously diagnosed the patient but the independent prescriber would still be responsible for the prescribing action. In other situations, the independent prescriber may be carrying out an assessment and be responsible for arriving at the diagnosis and treatment plan.

Writing the prescription

What constitutes a prescription? Nurses can prescribe medication on the inpatient prescription chart if the patient is in hospital. Nurses can also prescribe medication on outpatient slips or a prescription pad. When nurses prescribe on a pad, they will use FP10 prescriptions. These are pads that have the nurse's name and unique identification number on each page. A nurse seeing the patient, deciding on the medication and then advising a general practitioner to prescribe it through a letter or a phone call is not prescribing.

It is important that when a patient presents for service, other treatment options are considered. Nurse prescribers may wish to ensure that they have an established diagnosis and that the treatments proposed will be used within their licence preparation and dose range. Nurse prescribers also need to consider the wider implications of prescribing medication. It is worth restating that medication should be prescribed when all other reasonable nonpharmacological options have been considered. For some patients the prescription of medication helps to legitimise the sick role and gain attention for their emotional difficulties. This is why it is important that nurse prescribers consider why they are prescribing for their patient.

Terminating the supplementary and independent prescribing agreement

Some patients may be ideal at the start of the decision of a supplementary or independent prescribing framework but this may change for a host of reasons. Some patients may change in presentation and have unexplained symptoms, deviate from expected norm or develop side effects unfamiliar to the nurse. A frequent reason may be because the patient is moving from one area of care to the other, such as from hospital to home. The area of practice for nurse prescribers is not likely to pass domains of care.

A clinical management plan can be terminated at any time at the discretion of the psychiatrist or the nurse prescriber or the patient. Before this takes place, it is important that the prescribing role of the nurse is transferred back to the psychiatrist or the general practitioner. This transfer of care needs to be clear and a note made in the clinical record. It also suggests that the clinical management plan, if in a paper-based format, is cancelled and struck through and then filed in the patient's notes.

Training and the nurse-prescribing curriculum

In order for nurses to be eligible to prescribe medication, they need to undergo a statutory training programme run by the higher education institutions. The originator of these courses was the now-defunct Welsh National Board/English National Board, but with their dissolution, the Nursing & Midwifery Council took control of this area of training.

The training is 3–6 months long and includes 25 taught days in college with a further 12 days of supervised practice overseen by a designated supervising medical practitioner. The course is generic and includes topics such as consultation and prescribing in practice and, importantly, the governance arrangements surrounding the prescribing of medication.

The generic nature of the course leads onto a natural critique from the specialist branches of nursing, particularly mental health. Mental health nurses have found the pharmacology teaching sessions unhelpful for their mental health practice. This has probably contributed to implementation deficit as practitioners finish the course fully aware of the legal and professional issues to do with prescribing but to become aware of their significant gaps in knowledge.

This has led to various institutions and NHS trusts developing medication management training courses specifically for mental health nurses. The course run by University of Worcester is a 10-day (10-week) programme specifically designed to teach psychopharmacology. A wider course run by the Institute of

Table 2.4   Criteria to determine the appropriateness to train as a nurse prescriber

First-level nurse registered with the Nursing & Midwifery Council and 3 years post-registration clinical experience	Nurses must demonstrate this by showing the annotation on their Nursing & Midwifery Council records to their employer. The year preceding the joining of the course must be in their intended clinical setting to practice as an independent prescriber.
Able to study at Level 3	The course is set at graduate level with objective structured clinical examinations, case study material and a multiple-choice examination.
Designated supervising medical practitioner willing to provide 12-day learning in practice	This is mandatory and requires careful selection to ensure appropriate preparation. Nurses will find that this is the minimum requirement and extensive support is required post qualification.
Post where the nurse prescriber can prescribe and have access to a drug budget and, importantly, where nurse prescribing is a requirement for the post	Nurses need to be assured they can prescribe from a drug budget.
Employer honouring continuous professional development	Nurse prescribers will require constant access to training, supervision and mentoring post qualification, far more than the prescribing course can offer.

Psychiatry, London, encompasses not only psychopharmacology but also concordance techniques. Of late, universities themselves have developed specific mental health nurse-prescribing courses, which not only comprise the elements required to satisfy the Nursing & Midwifery Council but also applied psychopharmacology. This seems the natural way forward to enable nurses to prescribe medication.

Dissolved government in the UK has led to differing amounts of awards in universities for the same course. For example, the training for supplementary prescribing in England and Wales was awarded 30 CAT points at Level 3, whilst in Northern Ireland, 60 CAT points were awarded for the same training.

Part of the training programme is to have supervision and teaching from a designated medical supervising practitioner (the chosen psychiatrist). The role of the psychiatrist is to support and prepare the nurse through training (National Prescribing Centre 2005b). Psychiatrists attend a 1-day programme to support them in their role. In theory, the psychiatrist should facilitate learning in a supervised practice situation, thus enabling the trainee to think critically and apply theory to practice. The trainees are expected to carry out a structured clinical examination on patients under their care for their practice, which is monitored by the psychiatrist.

The reality for doctors and nurses may be somewhat different in terms of training and supervision experiences. Polar experiences range from the dedicated

Table 2.5 Issues to consider for the selection of designated supervising medical practitioner

Training and support for designated supervising medical practitioners	Psychiatrists should be encouraged to contact others who have supported nurses to be prescribers.
Should designated supervising medical practitioners be selected by the organisation and then accredited?	Not all doctors are suitable to supervise nurses given their views on new ways of working. In teams where nurse prescribing is required, job plans should identify the role of the psychiatrist to support nurse prescribers.
Why should psychiatrists carry out the role?	Add flexibility to the team and make better use of the resources by nurses and doctors.
Role of the designated supervising medical practitioner	Provide supervision and opportunities to increase competency. Nurses and doctors will find this becomes a regular feature post-qualification.

approach described above to a lacklustre approach from others. Organisations need to be careful in selecting the right doctors to be designated supervising medical practitioners. There has been no evaluation of what designated supervising medical practitioners think about their role (Table 2.5).

Patient group directions

Patient group directions are written instructions about the supply or administration of a named drug to a specific group of patients who may not be individually identified before presenting for treatment. They are legal documents that must be signed by the doctor, pharmacist and clinical governance lead. Each patient group direction must contain the date it comes into practice and the date of expiration (National Prescribing Centre 2004). Patient group directions can be developed for 80% of patient groups given the homogeneity of the diagnostic needs and treatment outcomes. To this end, it seems sensible for patient group directions to be written and used more extensively in service.

Patient group directions should be limited to situations where they offer an advantage to patients, obviously without compromising safety. Situations may arise when a large group of patients may require the same intervention. A good example is services for people with drug addiction or smoking cessation. Patient group directions may also be used when there may well be delays in service. For example, home treatment teams encounter people who are in distress and would provide them benefit from pharmacological interventions. A nurse can use a patient group direction to administer a single dose of olanzapine for aroused and agitated behaviour associated with schizophrenia (drug licensed for this use) (BNF 2008).

Guidance has been already established by the National Prescribing Centre (2004, 2005a), detailing how organisations can develop patient group directions for mental health.

(1) Patient group directions should be developed by a multidisciplinary group of staff including doctors, pharmacists and nurses.
(2) Drug and therapeutic committee should ratify the development of the patient group direction.
(3) The senior psychiatrist and senior pharmacist should formally sign off the patient group direction and should be involved in its development.

Policies to support implementation

The passing of legislation to enable nurses to prescribe medication is just one piece of the jigsaw for implementation. Government and professional organisations have been very keen to support implementation of mental health nurse prescribing and have sought to develop guidance to demonstrate how supplementary and independent prescribing can work. The National Prescribing Centre (2005a) carried out a review of the evidence behind mental health nurse prescribing. A survey of nurse directors in England highlighted areas where they thought supplementary prescribing should be implemented, namely assertive outreach teams and community mental health teams. This guidance has been helpful in refocusing the agenda for mental health practice. The guidance noted at the time that mental health NHS trusts in England had been disparate in their implementation of prescribing.

A second policy paper, this time led by the Department of Health, outlined what successful nurse prescribing projects would look like in mental health settings (DoH 2008d). There was an acknowledgement of the merits and demerits of supplementary and independent prescribing for certain practice settings. Important also was recognition of what factors or environmental conditions are required for mental health nurse prescribing to flourish. An example is how organisations had developed clinical governance to support role redesign and assurance of competency. The overall thrust of the document was a road map for implementation of nurse prescribing across a range of mental health settings.

In 2006, the Nursing & Midwifery Council (2006) published guidance for all nurses on the professional standards who are about to begin and who practice as a prescriber. They outline professional, ethical and legal requirements. Importantly, it is the employing organisations that are rightly charged with ensuring that nurse prescribers are appropriately managed and monitored, especially with regards to continuous professional development.

A year later, the Nursing & Midwifery Council published standards for qualified nursing staff for medicines management (Nursing & Midwifery Council 2007). Within this document, 26 standards are laid down about the responsibilities for those nurses who administer medication and those who prescribe it. Importantly, it covers how prescribing errors should be reported and subsequently managed. Essentially, nurse prescribers need to be continually mindful of their responsibilities but be honest and truthful with the patient and their organisation if they make an error. Reckless or malicious practice on the part of the prescriber would be a different situation.

Conclusion

In this chapter, the global expansion of nurse prescribing has been reviewed. Nurse prescribing is occurring in many developed and developing countries, implementation governed by issues of access to health services. Examples in Africa exemplify the health benefits that can occur for the local population by having nurses that can prescribe medication. The UK is a relatively new entrant into this new field but the challenges that have spurred it on have been the same. The introduction of nurse prescribing brings with it many challenges if the merits are to be realised, the first being how nurses can bring about new roles and improved medicines management. Primarily, the educational preparation for nurse prescribing requires a thorough revision in order for the future nursing workforce to deliver a modernised mental health service. This may result in new roles being developed such as nurse practitioners.

The development of nursing as a profession must occur for nurses to take on not only some of the advanced roles that come with nurse prescribing itself, but also the changing role that nurses will play when they have prescriptive authority. The development of nursing has at its heart the drive to deliver a competent and flexible workforce. In order for this to occur, changes to the way nurses are trained and prepared for the workforce will need to be adapted. Modernising Nursing Careers (DoH 2006e) and later workforce documents (DoH 2008c) set out a strategic vision of what types of roles nurses would be required to play in the future.

Chapter 3
The evidence base for nurse prescribing

Introduction

The advent of nurse prescribing is said to offer benefits for enhanced access to medicines and better use of nurses and doctors. However, there are worries about patient safety and the overall organisational governance arrangements, particularly independent nurse prescribing.

There have been a great deal of research enquiry into nurse prescribing in general and the conclusions are helpful within the broader context of mental health. However, it is the clues from mental health nurse-prescribing research where we will find the answers and solutions for the way forward, particularly problems in implementation. Development of the research material for mental health nurse prescribing will help to inform prescribing practice.

National and international studies demonstrate that nurse prescribing has become established into health services. The question to be considered in this chapter is whether nurse prescribing has led to improved access to medication, satisfaction with care, improved multidisciplinary team working and safety of prescribing activity.

What do clinicians think about nurse prescribing?

A large number of studies in the UK and the USA have focused on exploring the views of staff on the effects of nurse prescribing (Nolan *et al.* 2001; Hemingway 2004; Allsop *et al.* 2005; Jones 2007c,d; Jones *et al.* 2007; Jones 2008). Nolan *et al.* (2001) used a self-selecting sample of nurses who attended a 1-day conference on nurse prescribing. The main findings from this survey study indicate that psychiatric nurses were very keen to embrace prescriptive authority. A number of reasons were identified, such as the nature of the nurse–patient relationship that would allow greater access to, and monitoring of, medication. However, psychiatric nurses acknowledged the lack of education and training to support their current role in medication management and anxieties were expressed over extended prescriptive authority.

McCann & Baker (2002) looked at how the New South Wales nursing board extended the role of nurses into the domain of nurse practitioners. Part of the practitioner role involved prescriptive authority, but this was to be limited to prescribing for mental health problems. Respondents also argued in favour of clinical supervision and top-up training courses to support nurse prescribers in their role.

Views have been collected from pharmacists on the development of nurse prescribing. One study by Cooper *et al.* (2000) found that pharmacists had reservations about the competencies of nurse prescribers to prescribe contraception. When groups of professionals work together, professional differences become more apparent. It is interesting that mental health pharmacists who have been trained to be a prescriber do not actually practise when qualified. This has led to the suggestion that pharmacist time should be reserved for providing supervision of nurse prescribers.

Others have studied nurse perceptions in the USA, principally in the state of Colorado. Carr *et al.* (2002) found that psychiatric nurses were positive about prescriptive authority because it enabled them to spend more time with patients and treat the patients in a holistic fashion. This helped to reduce the amount of disjointed care within a very fragmented system. Findings from this study also indicated that nurses perceived the overall workload on medical staff would be reduced through nurse–physician collaboration and they would manage the large amount of routine care, leaving highly complicated care for the doctors to manage. However, there was also a perception that medical staff would be unsupportive of nurse prescribing because of the territorial claim to prescriptive privilege.

Jones (2006c,d) looked at what mental health nurses and psychiatrists thought about inpatient nurse prescribing within the context of supplementary prescribing. A focus group method was used with staff who worked in a psychiatric unit. The major conclusion from this research was that nurses and psychiatrists felt the relationship between the two professions was fundamental for supplementary prescribing to work effectively. Factors to develop the relationship included trust in the ability of the nurse to prescribe medication. A shared learning experience where the nurse and the psychiatrist together interviewed patients to construct a clinical management plan was also fundamental to develop relationships.

A further study by Jones (2008a) looked at the perception of nurses and psychiatrists about independent prescribing but this time for the broader family of mental health services, including adults, older people and substance misuse. A fairly hostile view was held about this development, primarily because of the distinct roles that nurses and psychiatrists have in diagnosis and control, perceived as it is, over patient care. Notwithstanding these concerns, the respondents were able to identify areas for development, primarily for independent prescribing nurses to work within defined clinical areas of expertise and with a defined group of medicines. These findings reflect the views of the Nursing & Midwifery Council (2006) where nurses should practise independent prescribing only within their area of competency.

Later studies carried out by Nolan & Bradley (2007) tried to find out what mental health nurses think about the factors that led them to undertake nurse-prescribing courses. Many mental health nurses spend considerable time in their posts advising doctors about starting medication or titrating medication. They saw the role of medication as an integral part of their role. Mental health nurses felt that nurse prescribing would lead to their better engagement with patients in terms of shared information and the time spent. They also felt that having prescriptive authority would help them to give their best in services. Two major points that one can take from the study are that mental health nurses interpreted the introduction of nurse prescribing to bring about a 'cost-cutting exercise', whilst the non-mental health respondents saw nurse prescribing as a way to reduce organisational fragmentation. This possibly indicates differences in how it can be implemented into services, in that much more positive views will come about if nurse prescribing is perceived as the latter.

One of the largest studies that have evaluated extended formulary independent nurse prescribing has been helpful to dispel some of the myths about nurse prescribing (Latter *et al.* 2007). A survey of 118 nurses who had undertaken the extended formulary nurse-prescribing course plus 10 case studies of practice settings were used as the unit of analysis. The majority of the sample were working in general practice or clinical settings attached to primary care. The most common conditions prescribed for were soft tissue injuries, skin conditions and family planning. Medical views of the nurse-prescribing activity were that the nurses were not always clinically appropriate and generally unable to note the appropriate details to back up the prescribing decision. Interestingly, the study demonstrated that the nurses held the view that they had become less dependent on doctors and nurse prescribing had improved the quality of patient care.

Grant *et al.* (2007) studied the views of staff when supplementary prescribing was introduced into a memory clinic for people with dementia. The study was small in that only seven members of the staff who were associated with the nurse-prescribing project were included. In terms of access, the staff reported that patients received a quicker and less interrupted service. Care was seen to be more total with less need to refer to the psychiatrist. This is a good outcome if patients can liaise with a single professional, receive an assessment and have their treatment. The memory clinic was seen as an ideal delivery vehicle to deliver nurse prescribing because of its consistent and clear approach. Advantages of prescribing within a memory clinic were seen both for patients to receive their care and in how care should be organised. The way professions should be used, and importantly reducing the difficulties in accessing psychiatrists, was also seen as a beneficiary of nurse prescribing, principally because patients were filtered off to nurses who could deliver a prescribing service.

Themes that have emerged from this research into nurses' perceptions of nurse prescribing include:

(1) differences in how supplementary and independent prescribing may benefit patients;
(2) improved job satisfaction and autonomy for nurses;
(3) ability to influence health care so that the patient receives person-centred care.

Interprofessional issues

The development of supplementary and independent nurse prescribing within the UK both have the potential to polarise the relationship between nurses and doctors. This is why it is important to evaluate the impact of nurse prescribing on the functioning of the team.

Howard & Greiner (1997) carried out a survey on mental health workers regarding prescriptive authority and noted a number of barriers, namely intraprofessional constraints and the inability of nonmedical staff to follow through on treatment decisions (i.e. admit to hospital). This may manifest as role confusion within clinical practice but also be linked to professional encroachment, power struggles and control exercised by one occupational group over another. Indeed, Kaas *et al.* (1998) found that nurses had difficulty in forming a collaborative relationship with their psychiatrist, which was one of the major barriers to nurses being granted prescriptive authority.

In a further study, Kaas *et al.* (2000) examined the characteristics and nature of the collaborative relationship between mental health clinical nurse specialists and doctors. They used a 34-item 5-point Likert questionnaire and examined returned forms from 49 nurses and 32 collaborating physicians. Satisfaction rates were high in that 75% of nurses and 84% of doctors reported being either satisfied or very satisfied with the relationship. Nurses and doctors who had more years of experience in practice and those with more experience in prescribing together tended to show higher levels of satisfaction. Psychiatrists in particular also benefited greatly in their ability to share caseload responsibilities with their collaborating nurses.

Prescriptive privileges may raise questions regarding the professional status of nurses. Nurses may also question the lack of financial compensation for the activity of prescribing, recognition by their peers and levels of autonomy in practice. Some have argued that nurses would also need to experience levels of support and supervision from their collaborating psychiatrist if nurse prescribing was to flourish (McCann & Hemingway 2003).

In the study by Jones *et al.* (2007), nurses and psychiatrists experienced an enhanced team effect in terms of skill, knowledge and practice by having a prescriber within the team. This has been supported by the fact that no safety concerns were noted in this study by nurses prescribing medication. Interestingly, there was an acknowledgement that prescribing errors could equally be made by doctors as well as by nurses.

Bradley & Nolan (2007) undertook a study to look at the early experiences of recently qualified nurse prescribers from a range of different disciplines (including mental health). It was readily acknowledged that nurse prescribing would lead to a change in the nursing role. Nurse prescribing was seen as more than just 'an add-on' to the nursing role, more of a fusion and development of the nursing profession. A key finding of this paper was the potential driver for nurse prescribers to integrate into the multidisciplinary team and the impact of a nurse prescriber on the dynamics of the team. Nurse prescribers, by the nature of their preparation and new understanding on medicines, will change the traditional medical hegemony of doctors being the perceived expert on drugs. They are positioning themselves as another voice in the team on how medication could be used. A recent survey comparing the views of nurses and psychiatrists to supplementary prescribing gives some interesting insights into professional differences on the value of nurse prescribing (Tomar *et al.* 2008). Nurses and psychiatrists were aware of supplementary prescribing. However, more nurses [compared to psychiatrists] were positive about the act of prescribing delivering a quicker access to medication and to improve patient care (Tomar *et al.* 2008).

A knock on effect of nurse prescribing is the challenge to traditional roles carried out by nurses and doctors. It is important that doctors are seen as collaborators in the nurse-prescribing initiative and not as a force to react against. Nurse prescribing will change the dynamics of how team rules are followed. The challenge is to use nurse prescribing as a force for good such as freeing up medical time. This may then support doctors to see how nurse prescribing could work further within the team (Bradley & Nolan 2007). Nurse prescribing must also be seen to enhance multidisciplinary team working as opposed to leading nurses to work in isolation from their colleagues.

Nurse prescribers may also bring about a greater interest in medicines management within the team. The wider nursing and multidisciplinary team also benefits, in turn, from having a nurse prescriber. Nurses can approach the nurse prescriber for advice on medication dosage and treatment effect. The experiences of nurse prescribing on the use of drugs will be helpful in presenting treatment options to patients.

It will be important for a deeper analysis on the nature of the relationship between the nurse and the doctor, to ensure that the collaborative agreement works well in practice. Moreover, research into the types of patients that would best be served by this new form of prescriptive authority would help to support long-term implementation.

Themes that have emerged from this research base include the following.

(1) Multiprofessional experience and understanding of nurse prescribing is underdeveloped and may differ between professional groups.
(2) Relationships between nurses and doctors become more positive over time.
(3) Changes in role boundaries between nurses and doctors occur when prescribing takes place in teams.

Outcomes for patients who have a nurse prescriber

Nurse prescribers on the whole believe that patients have faster access to service and improved understanding of their care through better information processes (Lewis-Evans & Jester 2004; While & Biggs 2004). Some areas of nursing, such as diabetic care, have demonstrated reduced hospital stay and reduced prescribing errors (Courtenay *et al.* 2007). The hard evidence for mental health nursing is less clear.

There is evidence that nurse-prescribing patterns of nurse practitioners are in line with general practitioners for certain diagnostic categories (Venning *et al.*

2000; Horrocks *et al.* 2002). Running *et al.* (2006) examined the prescribing patterns of nurse practitioners and physicians for back pain, musculoskeletal injury and bronchitis. Nurses generally prescribed fewer medicines than physicians for bronchitis and pain relief. A larger study looked at an evaluation of extended formulary independent prescribing and found that nurses stayed within their area of competency (Latter *et al.* 2005). This line of argument suggest that nurses can deliver services instead of general practitioners for certain conditions, and that nurses do not stray from their scope of competency, which begins to address concerns about patient safety. This has been supported by a political imperative that suggests suitably qualified nurses with extra training can take on 20% of the work carried out by general practitioners and junior medical staff (Wanless 2004).

Fisher & Vaughan-Cole (2003) examined similarities and differences in illness complexity of patients treated by nurse practitioners in comparison to psychiatrists within a large public health centre serving a population of just under a million. During a 1-year time frame, of 7251 patients, 76% had contact with either a nurse practitioner or a psychiatrist or both. Results demonstrated no significant differences in severity of patients treated by a nurse or a psychiatrist. However, patients treated by both a nurse practitioner and a psychiatrist were noted to be more severely ill. Nurse practitioners treated more people with axis 1 substance misuse disorder. For axis 2 disorders, nurse practitioners treated more patients diagnosed with a personality disorder.

However, a later study looked at this issue again and concluded with different results (Greenberg *et al.* 2006). The study looked at the proportion of patients who saw doctors and nurse prescribers in a Veterans Affairs hospital. This was a large study in that it captured the care of 767 920 patients who accessed service in 2002. The study indicated that patients who had a serious mental illness such as schizophrenia or mood disorder were more likely to see a doctor. The study concluded that nurse prescribers could not substitute doctors, although it is generally accepted that nurse prescribing was never about replacement of medical colleagues.

Fisher & Vaughan-Cole (2003) also examined case records of 120 random medication charts within the sample and found the total number of different medications prescribed was the same for nurses and psychiatrists, although psychiatrists prescribed different classes of antidepressant medications. The study also found that nurses spent more time with patients compared to a psychiatrist during a medication evaluation.

A further study from the USA looked at patients diagnosed with depression and their treatment by nurse prescribers and psychiatrists (Jacobs 2005). The treatment outcome was adherence to medication. In all 122 patients with depressive-type conditions were entered into the study. There was no difference in adherence rates if a psychiatrist or a nurse prescriber treated them. However, there were differences in that doctors prescribed more anxiolytic drugs. Doctors tended to spend less time with patients using therapy to augment psychotropic medication.

Issues that have emerged from this literature include the following.

(1) There is a view that nurse prescribing delivers equal, if not better, outcomes for patients.
(2) There is no evidence from the UK on whether mental health nurse prescribing makes any difference on patient outcomes.
(3) There are differences in the types of patients seen by nurse prescribers and doctors.

Views of patients on mental health nurse prescribing

One of the drivers for nurse prescribing is that nurses are able to develop therapeutic relationships with patients and use the amount of time they have in their clinical encounter to foster this. Research studies show that staff believes nurse prescribing lends itself to the social role that nurses hold in society and their ability to relate to patients (Grant *et al.* 2007). Given that assessment and diagnosis requires patients to be able to tell the history of their illness and expectations of past, present and future treatment, the interpersonal aspect of nurse prescribing becomes very important. As previously discussed in Chapter 1, some aspects of psychiatric nursing are not endowed with high levels of therapeutic engagement. However, the picture is changing as nurse prescribing demands high levels of purposeful engagement to be able to prescribe appropriately.

In the USA, care delivered by advanced practice nurses who prescribe medication has favourable outcomes in terms of acceptance by patients (Talley & Brooke 1992; Brooten *et al.* 2002). Interpreting this conclusion is difficult as patients may actually like to see the advanced practice nurse and may place higher value on this than on the prescribing activity. An Australian study examined the impact of unrestricted nurse prescribing (independent prescribing) for people with schizophrenia who received depot medication. Results were positive in favour of nurse prescribing (McCann & Clark 2008).

There have been a number of completed studies that chart the views of patients on nurse prescribing, for example, in primary care (Brooks *et al.* 2001). This has led to some researchers to look at what people think about nurse prescribing before they become ill. Berry *et al.* (2006) used an interesting method of posing to people the scenario of having a heart condition and its subsequent treatment. The study noted that people were generally unconcerned about the professional group of prescribing as long as they are trained and competent to prescribe for the condition. This probably reflects the changing focus in society about choice and a general scepticism about the medical profession in general.

In one of the early studies examining the effects of extended nurse prescribing, Luker *et al.* (1998) interviewed 148 patients being seen by practice nurses, district nurses and health visitors. Findings from this study demonstrated that patients were in favour of nurse prescribing in a number of ways. Patients identified the positive nature of the nurse–patient relationship, which enabled them to be more receptive to prescribing information. Patients felt that nurses gave them more time to discuss their problems, and treatment was found to be more accessible with over half of respondents preferring to be seen by a nurse as opposed to a doctor. Patients also perceived nurses to have unique areas of knowledge on treatment conditions. Luker *et al.* (1998) suggested that the unique social position of the nurse–patient relationship affected treatment preferences of patients in a positive way.

It is important to appreciate choice in how patients access medical care and how they wish their medical consultation to be conducted. For example, in one large general practitioner study, patients were asked to complete an agenda prior to the consultation. A number of interesting themes emerged: all patients had a specific question to ask the doctor, and of these, 60% of patients had a view on the cause of their problem. Similarly, 38% of patients had an explanation for their symptoms (McKinley & Middleton 1999). Clinical implications suggest that services need to engage with the user agenda but also modernise to offer patients choices in the type of professionals they see.

Harrison (2003) undertook a qualitative study on the views of psychiatric patients towards the development of nurse prescribing. Harrison found that mental health patients in the UK offered a cautious view on whether nurses had the required skill and knowledge to undertake the extended role and were concerned that diagnosis and treatment would displace the core nursing activities. Fundamental to psychiatric treatment is the nurse–patient relationship and any developments in prescriptive authority must ensure that interpersonal attributes such as trust, compassion and partnership working are not undermined.

Harrison's research was important to help set the context to nurse prescribing, but this study did not actually explore the reactions to people on the receiving end of mental health nurse prescribing. Jones *et al.* (2007) carried out a qualitative study on how mental health nurse prescribers, their patients and supervising psychiatrists viewed prescriptive authority. Patients valued the time nurses, in comparison to psychiatrists, gave them to discuss side effects of medication and also the choice offered in the type of medication.

There have been some interesting findings from patients treated by nurses who use independent prescriptive authority in a community-based setting (Wix 2007). Seventy-eight patients completed an 18-item questionnaire. Ninety-seven per cent of patients expressed the view that they had confidence in nurses prescribing their medication and access to treatment had improved. Interestingly, only 15% of patients thought the treatment they received from a nurse was the same as that received from a doctor. Reasons for this included more time for consultation to discuss the treatment. However, it is probably not just the time that is important. Most likely, the content of the consultation is different and includes more information about medication and side effects.

Studies are emerging on patients' experience or perception of prescribing, which needs to be an important part of a future research agenda (McCann & Clark 2008). It would therefore seem sensible to prioritise this area for evaluation from a number of practice settings, particularly to find out what aspects of nurse prescribing patients like the most. Further research is also required to assess the impact of nurse prescribing on the therapeutic relationship between the nurse and the patient. This would include assessing whether nurses who prescribe their medication do so in combination with psychological therapies. Again, firm evidence is required on the best ways to deliver nurse-prescribing interventions to suit patient needs.

Themes that have emerged from this research base include the following.

(1) Patients are more likely to be included in prescribing decisions.
(2) Patients are more likely to receive information about their diagnosis and treatment.
(3) It is unclear when patients would actually like to see their doctor.
(4) Patients like to have their medication prescribed by a nurse possibly because of a difference in the consultation style.

Medication management

One of the biggest drivers for nurse prescribing is the area of medicines management. However, perceived deficits in nurse's knowledge to prescribe medication have fuelled numerous research studies (King 2004; Leathard 2001; Otway 2002; Sodha *et al.* 2002). Medicines management covers more than just prescribing. However, an anxiety for policy planners and implementers of the approach is about the knowledge that nurses have on medication. Before the introduction of mental health nurse prescribing, academics have focused on knowledge gaps about medication and its side effects. There are commentaries about the ideal location of psychiatric nurses to use their medication administration skills and observation of side effects to best manage people, with safety being at the forefront of further treatment. Hence, research studies have looked at nurses' knowledge, or lack of it, in terms of medication.

Connected to prescriptive authority is the detection and management of adverse drug reactions within the psychiatric population. Nurses have been generally poor at assessing side effects (Bennett *et al.* 1995). Jordan *et al.* (2002) carried out a study to investigate the use of checklists in community teams for those patients attending for treatment. In this study, nurses using a checklist detected more adverse drug reactions compared to a control group (results probably affected by the Hawthorn effect). Problems identified by the experimental group were clearly impacting on the patient's quality of life and overall physical health. Clinical implications for nurses include a need for monitoring the reduction of health risk in patients for common problems such as movement disorders, weight gain and diabetes, all of which are strongly associated with medication-induced symptoms.

Further studies have examined the implications of informing patients about potential side effects of medication. For example, tardive dyskinesia (abnormal body movements) occurs in 20% of patients treated with antipsychotic medication. Chaplin & Kent (1998) carried out a control group study on the effectiveness of informing patients about the risks of developing tardive dyskinesia. Following a single educational session, patients acquired more knowledge compared to the control group with no effect on clinical outcome or noncompliance with medication, if given at the start of therapy. Patients also began to appreciate nurses discussing their adverse drug reactions and hence reducing the health burden and improving medication concordance.

There have been studies that have looked at training mental health nurse prescribers in medication management and advanced psychopharmacology (Gray *et al.* 2004, Jones *et al.* 2007). Jones (2007) used a small sample of mental health nurse prescribers and tested their knowledge before and after the training. Following the training, mental health nurses demonstrated an increase in their knowledge base on depression, schizophrenia and bipolar disorder, which reached levels of significance. Findings from this study demonstrated a number of interesting points. First, baseline scores on knowledge were low and thus indicated a need for training. Second, gains in knowledge were achievable through a short focused course. Third, it was unclear how durable the training was over time and whether a more knowledgeable practitioner led to an increase in prescribing practice.

Two key issues that have come out of medication management research are the following.

(1) Nurse prescribers have deficits in knowledge but can acquire advanced pharmacological knowledge.
(2) Informing patients about side effects is important.

Implementation deficit research

Within the overall modernisation of health care, it is important to understand the enhancing and hindering factors for nurse prescribing. Studies looking at district nurses and health visitors who prescribe medication noted the rate and diffusion of prescribing to be variable across different sites (Luker *et al.* 1997; While & Biggs 2004; Hall *et al.* 2006). A large UK survey was carried out by Courtenay & Carey (2007) into a Nursing & Midwifery Council database of nurse prescribers (25% of all prescribers); 68% of independent nurse prescribers noted difficulties accessing a prescription pad and agreements to use a prescription pad. Supplementary prescribing nurses (54%) experienced problems in using the clinical management plan and the amount of time to write it. Integral to this is being able to contact a doctor to collaborate in the agreement.

An important area for mental health nurse prescribing is how far the approach has been implemented. Nurses from all backgrounds of nursing, notably community nursing (Hall *et al.* 2006) and mental health nursing (Bradley *et al.* 2005), acknowledge that supplementary prescribing is a worthwhile intervention. However, there are many organisational barriers to limit implementation. One notable problem in examining this area for the UK is that of the devolved countries and no survey being conducted to gather data on this.

Perhaps it is the characteristics of nurse prescribers and where they work that affect implementation. Campbell *et al.* (1998) carried out a survey of US psychiatric nurse prescribers and found that the majority of them worked in outpatient settings. Later, Talley & Richens (2001) examined the characteristics of US psychiatric nurse practitioners in those states that allowed prescriptive authority. A convenience sample of 88 nurse practitioners indicated that nurses had been prescribing medication for just over 4 years, although in those states with a history of prescribing, nurses had a longer duration; 38.6% of nurse practitioners worked in a community setting, 23.9% worked in independent practice and less than 15% worked in an inpatient setting. The mean number of patients seen per day was 7.98. Nurses also perceived their prescriptive trends to be similar to that of a psychiatrist, although 41.3% saw their practice to be more careful in the medication they prescribed. Very few of the nurses had 'admission privileges' resulting in the patient being referred to the emergency room if inpatient treatment was required.

Predominantly, research on collecting views on mental health nurse prescribing has been carried out in England. Gray *et al.* (2005) conducted a survey on implementation of supplementary nurse prescribing by asking executive nurses in England to report on the number of nurses who were trained and were practising as a nurse prescriber. Just over half of all trusts responded and so the findings were fairly indicative of prescribing practice. According to this survey, there were approximately two mental health nurses per trust who had completed the training. Of interest, the report indicated that community mental health teams had the maximum support for implementation, whilst inpatient care had the least. When this survey was completed, 66% of executive nurses did not think that psychiatrists had been adequately prepared to supervise or mentor nursing staff to carry out the supplementary prescribing role.

It is the gap in knowledge, principally on psychopharmacology, which has led to implementation deficit for some nurse prescribers. Skingsley *et al.* (2006) noted that the generic basis of the nurse-prescribing course leads mental health nurses to feel bereft of knowledge upon completion.

Although not looking specifically at mental health, an interesting study by Courtenay & Carey (2008) looked at the implementation of independent and supplementary prescribing. A national postal survey was used coupled with a case study of practice. For independent prescribing, the largest reported problem hindering implementation was restriction in local arrangements enabling nurses to prescribe (66%) followed by the difficulty in generating computer prescriptions (61%). Much less problems were related to lack of knowledge, peer support or support from medical staff. So in this sense, implementation appears to be one of organisational nature. For supplementary prescribing, difficulties related to the implementation of the clinical management plan coupled with local restrictions.

A second study worthy of inclusion was carried out by Ryan-Wooley *et al.* (2007). This study was a survey of 2252 Macmillan nurses (palliative care) in the UK. Nurse prescribers (*n*=203) were critical about the quality of medical supervision and training to enable them to be a prescriber. This was not helped by the course content being poorly correlated to palliative care (a feature similar to mental health). There was a general view that patients would not wish Macmillan nurses to be independent prescribers because of the perceived safety of prescribing. These factors hampered the take-up of nurse prescribing in this specialised area of nursing.

A particular problem that emerges from the nurse-prescribing implementation research is what type of patient would be suitable for nurse prescribing. Nurse prescribing may not be suitable for all patients, as some patients may need to see the psychiatrist for a review of unexplained symptoms and complex medical issues. Some studies have attempted to develop criteria to differentiate severe cases from those that could be seen by a nurse prescriber (Fisher & Vaughan-Cole 2003). This type of research is required for the UK.

Three key issues that have come from research on implementation deficit are as follows:.

(1) Take-up of prescribing has been slow in mental health.
(2) Not all clinical areas are deemed appropriate for prescribing to take place.
(3) Further research needs to be carried out on the applicability of independent prescribing for mental health settings.

Future research

The evidence base for nurse prescribing is just emerging, but what there is demonstrates support from organisations, nurses, doctors and service users. It is vital that new forms of interventions and service models receive thorough evaluation and include patient experiences and coverage of patient safety and effectiveness. As discussed previously, both qualitative and quantitative approaches have been used to explore the perceptions held by staff and patients towards nurse prescribing. Research in the USA has looked at the types of patients seen by nurses and doctors and touched on the relationships between nurses and doctors.

A word must be said about the quality of the research. Latter & Courtenay (2004) carried out a review of the research designs used to test nurse prescribing in the UK and concluded that the majority of studies were limited to self-report designs with limited 'generalisability' of research findings to the myriad of practice settings. Although their review was much wider than mental health, this conclusion covers mental health. Therefore, one must be cautious in saying that a robust evidence base supports mental health nurse prescribing.

A primary focus of research should be to collect attitudes and aspirations to use supplementary prescribing within the different service models. Acute psychiatric units would be a suitable setting, given the large numbers of patients seen and the potential for shared decision making with nursing staff. Patients' views should guide service development with the aim of increasing involvement and concordance in treatment decisions. Central to any prescriptive model will be the relationship between the nurse and the doctor. Certain factors to be considered include how nurses and doctors seek a collaborative relationship

(National Prescribing Centre 2003). An important research question would be how patients are deemed appropriate for a supplementary and independent prescribing relationship.

Useful research enquiry could be directed at finding out differences, if any, in what nurses and doctors prescribe. This is useful research for two reasons. The first is to make sure that nurses are prescribing drugs that are in line with established best practice. The caveat to this, however, is to bear in mind that the quality of medical prescribing in psychiatry is less than adequate (NPSA 2006; Healthcare Commission 2007b). The second is to see whether nurses use nonpharmacological intervention as a substitute for drug therapy. There is a general concern that patients have too much access to medication and nurses may contribute to this.

When we look at what is required for nurses to prescribe competently, the area of diagnosis comes into question. Under supplementary prescribing, the nurses do not need to arrive at a diagnosis because the doctor does it for them. With independent prescribing, this is entirely different, as nurses formulate their own diagnosis based on their assessment. This has driven some scholarly critique on the value of nurses carrying out a diagnostic interview to arrive at their formulation for treatment. The views of nurses on this form of activity remain a fertile ground for research.

A question that is considered by some is what is going on in the mind of the nurse prescribers when they prescribe medication. Is the decision-making process the same for doctors or do they take into consideration other factors? It is surprising that very little has been written on this important point because relational research between patients and nurses quite clearly demonstrates that social interaction is different and comes out of a prescribing decision-making process.

Future studies need to further demonstrate that nurse prescribing is as safe as usual prescribing patterns and can improve the prescribing carried out by doctors. Clinical governance structures around patient safety have been omitted from previous research.

Conclusion

The evidence base for mental health nurse prescribing is emerging. Notwithstanding the methodological flaws of the research studies, they outline three headline points.

First, nurse prescribing is seen as a good outcome for the profession. Nurses think that they are able and in a position to influence patients to take their medication. Nurse prescribing furthers this position.

Second, nurse prescribing is seen as a driver to modernise nursing, medical and allied health professions. Nurse prescribing has been heralded as the beat of the healthcare artery in the quest to transform services. Nurse prescribing provides opportunities to enable nurses to take up clinical positions; but would they be able to do the role any better than psychiatrists? There have been no head-to-head studies in the UK.

Third and the most important is the knowledge gap between the desire to prescribe and having the relevant knowledge to practise safely and to the limits that are afforded by independent prescribing. More work is required on this area to ensure nurses can be taught the relevant aspects of medical practice within their defined areas of competency.

In order for nurse prescribing to be seen as a legitimate activity, its outcomes must be clear. It needs to be verified that it is a safe and cost-effective alternative to patients seeing doctors. Patients must be satisfied with the care they receive. Access to service must be demonstrably better than the referral waiting list quagmire we have now.

Chapter 4
How to get nurse prescribing to work safely

Introduction

It must be remembered that nurse prescribing is a new and, at times, radical departure from usual ways of working. Organisations have started to train key nursing staff, and lessons have been learnt along the way to support future implementation. In order for organisations to allow nurse prescribers to work, systems must be in place that protect the public, organisation and nurse prescribers themselves.

The aim of this chapter is to discuss practical ways in which organisations can support the development of nurse prescribing. There are a host of reasons why organisations are not involved in the initiative but these can be overcome if nurses approach them with their organisations in a logical and concerted fashion.

This chapter also discusses how nurses can progress from being a supplementary prescriber to an independent prescriber. Certain steps are outlined that can support competency achievement. It is important for a nurse to work as a safe prescriber and the chapter will cover areas such as managing adverse drug events and drug errors.

Reasons why nurses are not prescribing

National and international reviews of nurse prescribing identify that nurses are generally satisfied with their prescribing roles. However, there are barriers to these roles, which include delays in actually being allowed to prescribe and, in some instances, obtaining a prescription pad. This chapter will not only cover the various facets to this 'implementation deficit' but also discuss ways in which nurses and doctors can overcome the inertia that is so evident in our organisations.

Lack of organisational planning

A major factor affecting many nurses is that the organisation has simply not invested time and energy into thinking how nurse prescribing can help patients. Some aspects of mental health care may have been missed off the radar in terms of local planning arrangements or hasty decisions made about the difficulties or supposed inappropriate use of prescribing. For example, some organisations may be following the lead from the National Prescribing Centre (2005) and hence may not implement prescribing in inpatient areas.

Access to the pad

Restrictions and difficulties in getting hold of a prescription pad has been reported in the literature (Fisher 2005; Hall *et al.* 2006). It is obvious that nurses cannot prescribe unless they can have access to a prescription chart as used in hospitals, or to a pad or an electronic prescribing system. There have been situations where nurses have not been able to access prescription pads and where nurses have had to wait several months for them to arrive. Specifically for drug and alcohol services, pads are specific for prescribing morphine. In Wales, this has been a particular problem for some nurse prescribers who wish to prescribe controlled drugs. Presently, there is no stationery that can be used by a nurse prescriber for controlled drugs. Waiting for months for the prescription pad may lead to some nurses forgetting their prescribing skills or allowing doubt to creep in and hence stifle implementation.

There is a particular problem when nurse prescribers move to other organisations and then need to wait and enlist to get their pads. They find that they have to explain their roles and their prescribing practices to a whole set of new clinicians who may be unfamiliar with prescribing. This is also the case for the local pharmacy staff who may be unfamiliar with the signature of the nurse prescriber.

Nurses who interface with primary care are likely to work alongside general practitioners who prescribe electronically. Now it would seem quite a simple task for the primary care organisation to register nurses to use this electronic method. However, problems arise where this is simply not happening.

Nurse prescribers may also face difficulties in being able to access computer-generated prescriptions, which are becoming the norm in general practitioner surgeries across the UK. The problems appear to be local restrictions on the part of primary care organisations to allow nurses to register to prescribe on this system (Hall *et al.* 2006).

General practitioners are averse to nurses writing handwritten prescriptions. This organisational problem will also manifest in nurses being unable to share access to the patient record. Understandably, nurses will not prescribe medication for patients when they have an incomplete medical history.

Going up the ladder

It is true to say that the early cohorts of nurses who went on for the prescribing course were bright aspiring nurses. Many of them have not prescribed because they have gone onto higher positions that have simply taken them away from clinical contact. There are other nurses who have prescribed but relinquished this responsibility when they gained managerial and non-clinical positions.

Administrative burden

It can be argued that supplementary prescribing burdens the process of psychiatric care with unnecessary paperwork. Nurses spend lots of time carrying out paperwork not directly related to care tasks, and implementation of the clinical management plan was one of the barriers that hampered prescribing (Lewis-Evans & Jester 2004; Courtenay & Carey 2008). The practicalities of completing the clinical management plan and then meeting the psychiatrist and the patient to sign it results in delayed time. Sometimes it is simply easier for the nurse to have a trainee doctor prescribe medication than to go through the process of writing a clinical management plan.

Independent prescribing does not require the bureaucracy of a clinical management plan. Good medicines management would still require a medication care plan and this has been used to good effect in inpatient care by independent nurse prescribers (Jones 2008).

Working in roles where prescribing is not required

There is emerging evidence suggesting that nurses have been trained to be employed in roles that do not require the nurse prescribing skills, for example nurses working in community mental health teams. It seems illogical for nurses to take on prescribing responsibility for large groups of patients when in fact this prescribing can be and should be managed in primary care. There are a small group of people who require dose titration such as clozapine management or switching from one medicine to another. An example is of a patient who started on aripiprazole [licensed for the treatment of bipolar disorder (BNF 2008)] and required close monitoring for further dose titration when he or she was discharged by the home treatment team. In these circumstances, it is appropriate for a nurse to oversee this as a supplementary or independent prescriber.

Mental health consultation is vast in primary care and constitutes 25% of workflow in general practitioner surgeries (Goldberg & Huxley 1992). Common mental health problems such as depression and anxiety may require a pharmacological intervention. Mental health nurses who work at the primary care interface may be best placed to assess and treat the patient; if they do so, then only it is right and proper that they prescribe the medication. However, the practice of nurses working in different organisations with different rules prevents this reality from occurring.

One must also discuss the systems of care. The way we organise our teams is not dependent on nurse practitioners with prescriptive authority. By and large, teams are organised around the doctors, as they are the ones that can prescribe medication. This probably explains why it is so difficult to implement nurse prescribing.

The reality for most services is that the consultant psychiatrist does not write many prescriptions because prescribing is done by the general practitioner. In practice, the consultant psychiatrist writes to the general practitioners and advises them about medication changes. This may result in a delay if the letter is not faxed to the general practitioner and followed up by the nurse to prompt the action forward. This situation also occurs for community nurses where they may offer advice to the general practitioner about the presentation and medication. This inevitably leads to a situation where the system does not require the nurse or the psychiatrist to prescribe.

Reduced level of prescribing

If clinicians are going to prescribe medication then they need to be proficient with this new skill. Early implementation research demonstrates that very little nurse prescribing actually goes on in clinical practice (Gray *et al.* 2005). A Healthcare Commission (2007b) report on prescribing in mental health supports this conclusion. Only 43% of nurse prescribers stated that they prescribed on a weekly basis. This could be because of the lack of opportunity to prescribe through poor service contact. One-third of the trusts did not have supporting policy to underpin nurse prescribing. It seems ludicrous to allow nurses who prescribe infrequently to actually prescribe at all. Infrequent prescribing activity should not be confused with not prescribing. Not prescribing medication, on the other hand, is when the nurse has consulted the patient and decided to make no changes to medication. The two scenarios are different.

Knowledge

Chapter 5 will discuss the need for robust medicines management and training in mental state examination skills, although a barrier to implementation is that some doctors and nurses hold the belief that experience in the formulation of a diagnosis for complex pathology requires grounding in the natural sciences. Training in physiology, biochemistry, molecular biology, pathology and pharmacology is reserved for clinicians trained in medicine. Nurse training covers only a slight portion of these areas. There are some advocates in the medical profession who cannot see why nurses cannot learn to take on the diagnosis of complex pathology provided they are given the training and supervision (Siriwardena 2006). The position argued brings out two points. The first is that nurse prescribers may be trying to operate in a team where other clinical staff hold inferior views on the ability of the nurse prescriber to prescribe effectively and safely. The second problem is that the nurse may become acutely aware of their training gap and never prescribe.

However, a reality for nursing – one that must be contended with – is that diagnosis is not a routine aspect of nurse training. However, diagnosis and formulation is essential for nurses to prescribe medication. The challenge is for the process of arriving at a diagnosis to become part of nurse education.

The National Prescribing Centre (2005a) recommends that it may be beneficial for nurses to attend a medication management course before either starting or completing the prescribing course, for the full benefits of prescriptive privileges to be realised. However, this is reliant on organisations having access to accredited courses that will actually provide nurses with the right course content to assist in the delivery of medicines management.

Access to continuous professional development

With regard to feeling insecure in knowledge about disease and how drugs work we need to ensure that continuous professional development is in place and regularly attended. Organisations may employ nurses who do not have sufficient resources to enable them to access supervision and training on a regular basis. Junior doctors and psychiatrists have weekly half-day sessions devoted to audit, research and case conferences to cover the areas required for professional development. Organisations lack robust arrangements for nurses to feel confident to take on the huge responsibility of independent prescribing.

Attitudes of nursing staff within organisations

In Chapter 1, the tensions and opportunities that have come up through the expansion of psychiatric nursing into community settings have been laid out. It is our historical heritage that is both a driver and a constraint in moving the nurse-prescribing initiative forward.

It is evident that two schools of thought have an impact on the successful adoption of nurse prescribing. In the first, nurse prescribing is seen as a natural development of the profession in response to technological, cultural and societal changes. Mental health nurses are seen as the natural leaders to take on aspects of diagnosis and medicines management. It seems that if nurse leaders and change agents hold these views, nurse prescribing is likely to flourish.

The other school of thought is that nurse prescribing is an attempt by medicine and the government to 'medicalise' the role of psychiatric nurses. Advocates of this viewpoint believe that psychiatric nurses are there to support and advocate for and with patients when they are under the medical gaze. The danger is that the nurse who independently prescribes medication will be seen as the bargain basement doctor and would ill serve patients.

A further tension that gets played out in discussion is the traditional role of the nurse as a direct 'caregiver' as opposed to a 'treatment provider'. Nursing prides itself and is stereotyped in the media as the profession that provides care. Nurse prescribing is sometimes pitted against this conception. Statements are made that if you are a nurse prescriber then you lose the caring side of a nurse' traditional role. If nursing is to survive, it needs to come out of its traditional remit of trying to live up to its caricatures of providing the 'human touch' and 'caring'. Other health and social care professions also lay claim to these attributes. The reality also is that nurses do far more and are paid to provide services that go beyond the caring role.

Closer ties between nursing and medical staff also hinder implementation. Nurse-prescribing legislation and local policy guidance stipulate that psychiatrists must supervise nurses and check their competency (DoH 2006b). Nursing staff have fought long and hard for separation of their duties from medical staff. They forget the reality that health care is a continuum where medical and nursing staff work side by side and have done so for decades. However, nurses may reject nurse prescribing because of the supervision and oversight by medical staff.

Balancing where the profession has come from and where it is going needs to be worked through in order for nurses to play their part in the modern theatre of health care. Nurse prescribing does challenge the role of what nurses do and what doctors do. Nurses do need to respond to the key drivers and lead the way in meeting the challenges that now face the health service. The key is for nurses to respond but without throwing the baby out with the bathwater and to not lose the essential elements of what nurses do.

Remuneration

The majority of the NHS budget is spent on staff pay, leading to the drive to find more cost-effective ways to deliver services. There have been changes to the remuneration system for nurses through agenda for change. The knowledge skills framework provides a mechanism through which terms and conditions can be changed to take effect of new roles. Presently, many nurses are not specifically remunerated for their nurse-prescribing activity and this is clearly a barrier to implementation.

It is unclear how the modernised pay structure for nursing staff will reward those nurses who take on extended roles. The obvious question is why nurses should take on extra responsibilities for no increase in pay. This may explain why some nurses do not prescribe, although remuneration does not factor highly in many reported findings.

Independent prescribing is an extended role encompassing diagnosis and formulation. It seems unrealistic to expect nurses to undertake an independent prescribing role without remuneration. It is more likely that services will be reconfigured so that nurses with independent prescriptive authority can work to best meet the needs of patients.

Fear of litigation

When the reader takes on board the legal responsibilities of nurse prescribing, it will obviously lead to a reflection on one's own vulnerabilities. Nurse prescribers will have been subject to various lectures on vicarious liability and will be fully aware of where their professional liability starts and ends with nurse prescribing. Nurses need to feel supportive within this legal context. Recent DoH plans to force nurses to take out indemnity insurance will worsen the fear of litigation. However, the reality of the situation is that with greater autonomy comes responsibility. Nurses practicing in ways that cover diagnosis and treatment will bring them into situations where they may be subject to legal action if untoward events occur. Nurses may well stray into areas where they carry out actions beyond their scope of competency. Fear of litigation is a reality and will prevent nurses from taking on prescribing responsibilities.

Unstable teams

We have all worked in teams where focus and clear team cohesion is absent. For those nurses wishing to start nurse prescribing, this can be a disastrous bedrock to start from. Undoubtedly, nurse prescribing requires a stable staff mix, particularly the role of the consultant psychiatrist.

It is not just psychiatrists who may be vetoed for their lack of suitability. Nurse prescribers may join the team from other teams. It seems unlikely that a psychiatrist would inherit a nurse prescriber and then develop a collaborative relationship without a prior 'settling in' period.

Wrong people put forward

Guidance has been put forward listing the necessary requirements for suitable entry to the course for the nurse and attributes required for the psychiatrist. It seems that organisations have simply agreed with these without careful thought. The reality is that not all doctors or nurses are suited to this new way of working. It is also likely that the wrong people have been put forward for the training. This, to some degree, was inevitable given the novelty appeal of nurse prescribing when it was first launched. Time is needed for the numbers of appropriate people to build up in the system.

Access to the same patient record

A real need for nurse prescribers is to have access to the shared medical record. Nurse prescribing is reliant on an iterative continuous assessment process. Assessment and formulation go hand in hand. Nurses must refer to the patient record in order for informed prescribing decisions to be made. Some clinicians may work in teams that are displaced from the central patient record. This becomes a cause for concern for medical staff who supervises nurse prescribers.

Making nurse prescribing happen

Individuals and organisations have taken a number of routes to adopt nurse prescribing. Some of them are reviewed here. Not all will work because the context will be different, particularly for NHS care and independent care.

Understand organisational anxiety

Clinical governance is a framework that allows organisations to be assured that practice is safe and effective. In today's climate, the chief executive of NHS trusts in the UK is accountable for the quality of care given to patients. Nurses need to be aware that clinical governance and safety dominates trust board discussion. Clinical governance can therefore be seen as a barrier to implementation. Nurse prescribers need to understand how organisations think about risk and to communicate the complexity of nurse prescribing in simple terms. The objective is to stop organisations from getting stuck or paralysed about what may go wrong with extending nursing practice into the realm of non-medical prescribing. Nurses can do this by:

(1) being clear of national and worldwide policy and practice;
(2) using examples of application to single disease areas;
(3) understanding how risk has been minimised by nurse prescribing;
(4) being clear about the local risks of implementation.

Organisations have approached nurse prescribing by asking the nurse prescriber to write a risk assessment on the parameters of prescribing practice. The parameters of what can be prescribed are agreed between the manager, prescriber and clinical lead. This helps to limit the anxieties about 'nurses running off with the British National Formulary'. In some organisations, such protocols are also overseen by drug and therapeutics committees so that they are aware of the medicines being prescribed by nurses.

   To help manage anxiety, organisations should know who has prescriptive authority. Organisations tend to do this by maintaining a central database, which includes notification of Nursing & Midwifery Council entry for prescriptive authority. Senior nurses would be correctly concerned if they could not account for who has prescriptive authority and the authority of issuing prescription pads. The more nurse prescribers can think and articulate over arching clinical governance arrangements, the more likely it will be for organisations to allow them to prescribe.

Trust board 'buy-in'

Nurses who hold influential positions should be lobbied to bring about new roles and new systems to support nurse prescribers. It is really important that your nurse executive is aware of the practical reality of nurse prescribing. They will have previously responded to the policy imperative but will be stuck at the implementation stage. You may wish to unplug this stoppage by sending in examples of where nurse prescribing is working and what policies have been developed to support nurse prescribing at the implementation stage.

   Implementation of nurse prescribing must be focused on nurse leadership at board level. One of the most powerful ways to bring about board decision making is patient experience. Nurses need to demonstrate how patients will receive a quicker higher quality of service from a nurse who can prescribe medication.

   Engaging key medical staff is vital for successful implementation. Nurse prescribing is not just about giving out tablets. Nurse prescribing is tied up with service redesign and role change. Having senior medical staff buy in is essential so that the passage of change can be seen as acceptable. Strategies should demonstrate how the skills and expertise of medical staff can be enhanced by showing them how suitably trained nursing staff can competently assist them in managing their flow of work.

For those nurses who wish to prescribe medication, full support would be required from their medical supervisor and the lead consultant for the service. The budding nurse prescriber needs to convince them of the merits of the approach. One way for this enthusiasm to come across is to familiarise oneself with local formularies and how the drugs can be used to better effect through a nurse-prescribing process. If nurse prescribing is being put forward in a new area, it is unlikely to take place if it is left to medical staff.

Nurse prescribers need to adopt the strategy of persuading a few of the doctors in the organisation. More doctors will follow when a lead clinician, such as the clinical director, takes the lead or offers no obstruction.

Nurses and managers need to demonstrate that nurse prescribing is not just about giving nurses status, but about improving care for patients. Psychiatrists should be involved in how models of service can improve so that they are not seen as 'being done to'.

Each organisation will have a non-medical prescribing lead. The prescribing enthusiast needs to identify and link in with this person and involve him or her in the reasons why nurse prescribing will improve patient care.

Establish a nurse-prescribing steering group

Clinicians who are trained to prescribe and who are then prescribing require a forum to discuss and share experiences. Such forums can be helpful to get the initiative going. However, the green shoots of implementation need to be nourished by having a group of nurse prescribers who actually practise their skills. They require a different type of support, as all nurse prescribers know, there is a difference in talking about prescribing and the realities of putting pen to the prescription pad.

If a prescribing group does meet in your trust, nurse prescribers should meet with their peer nurse prescribers so that they can discuss how their peers are prescribing medication within their own particular areas. Nurse prescribing develops differently for different parts of mental health services. Peer support is fundamental to challenge the nurse prescriber to think much more broadly about their prescribing role within a safe environment.

New ways of working vision

All organisations adapt and change to service pressure. Key clinical champions must at every opportunity highlight the opportunities that may emerge with nurse prescribing. It must be viewed as a tool or the grease to ease in change and unplug gaps. Nurses should be able to clearly articulate which clinical areas would benefit from nurse prescribing and to develop a communication plan to inform patient and clinical and managerial layers in the organisation. Nurse prescribing will not occur without a 'new ways of working' vision.

There are a number of initiatives that have supported new ways of working such as the 'refocusing project' (Bowles & Jones 2005) and 'creating capable teams' (DoH 2007b). The aim of these initiatives is to bring about different ways of working by maximising the roles and skills of the team(s). Areas to consider within these exercises include:

(1) establishing the role and purpose of the team;
(2) selecting the mechanism for system redesign;
(3) identifying how education and training can bring about new roles;
(4) identifying how does the role of the prescriber interface with other workplace partners

The nature of nursing work is to spend lots of time with patients. Nurses pride themselves on understanding the social world of patients, their family backgrounds and personal needs. Connecting the agenda of medicines management, mental state examination and overall case management adds a different dimension to health care. Nurses who are able to offer this combination of skills would be more attractive to employers that embrace a socially inclusive model of care. The point is for nurse prescribers to offer something different to the patient and add value to the business of the organisation.

The burden of disease that occurs with demographic shifts calls for a different way of informing patients about how to manage and treat their illnesses. Nursing staff who embrace a health-promoting philosophy whilst also undertaking necessary prescribing duties will support new ways of working.

Healthcare is fragmented with aspects of the care and treatment of the patient's problem distributed to different professionals working within the same team and in different teams. This is unavoidable for some aspects of care. However, with further training, aspects of care can be consolidated so that professionals can deliver more of the care. The end game would be for nurse prescribers to deliver packages of care. Nurse prescribing is a skill set that helps service providers to think about how this may happen.

Trust awareness sessions

It is helpful to have meetings that spell out the broad principles of nurse prescribing. You may find it helpful to invite your clinical lead to chair the session and to have external speakers who have implemented nurse prescribing. The aim is to raise awareness of the point that debate about nurse prescribing has progressed into implementation and how prescriptive authority can inform service redesign.

Identify enthusiasts and spread the word

Nurse prescribing will not happen unless you have enthusiastic and competent senior clinicians who actually prescribe in practice. Such individuals should be carefully selected, trained and promoted to take on leadership roles. The aim should be to spread the positive gospel about nurse prescribing and dispel myths about safety in the minds of people who could block nurse prescribing. Potential enthusiasts may be:

(1) clinical and medical directors;
(2) collaborating psychiatrists;
(3) non-medical prescribing leads;
(4) new ways of working champions.

Organisations and individuals need to accept that nurse prescribing is part of a long game. Quick wins will be achieved. The reality, however, is that widespread dissemination is difficult. Key opinion leaders in your organisation should develop examples of good practice and have them published in trust or organisational briefing letters. They serve as a passive tool to introduce nurse prescribing that some clinicians may find a threat.

Get yourself a good mentor

Psychiatrists are highly trained and skilled in psychopathology and treatment. Nurse prescribers need to soak up this knowledge in abundance. It makes people feel valued and appreciated when they are asked for help and when they impart information to willing recipients. The reality also is that nurse prescribers need this knowledge to improve their clinical skills. Organisations will also be more willing to take down some of the barriers when they see a team approach that has competent doctors to oversee implementation.

In order for nurses to progress in their prescribing careers, it is important for the psychiatrist to be aware of the levels of competency that nurses possess. This will only occur when a nurse and a psychiatrist work together as part of a team. It seems impossible to imagine a situation where a psychiatrist would enter into a collaborative relationship with a nurse prescriber whom he or she does not know. It is up to the nurse prescriber to foster the relationship with the psychiatrist to gather experience and extend his or her competence. The payoff for the psychiatrists may be their patients receiving a better overall management of their care from a nurse prescriber. However, nurse prescribers also need to be aware of the amount of time required from the psychiatrist to prepare them in their role (Table 4.1).

Avoid working in isolation

Nurse prescribing requires continuous professional development and exposure to your own and other people's practice. The most important advice is to develop relationships with not only your mentoring psychiatrist but also other doctors and nurse prescribers. Linking in with current audit practice on what medication is being prescribed and prescribing trends in your area will help illuminate prescribing practice that is off kilter.

Table 4.1   Attributes of a successful mentor

Experienced in psychiatry	Look for doctors who have been trained for more than 3 years post specialist training.
Leadership	Look for doctors who have worked on projects for the organisation and have demonstrated that they can deliver on organisational objectives. This is most likely to carry 'organisational weight' when trying to get prescribing implemented within your own organisation.
Supervision and teaching	You need a doctor who can impart information without making you feel stupid or incompetent. Avoid doctors who 'get off' on being the one with all the knowledge. You need information about pathology and drugs so that you can make your own decisions.
Close clinical association	It seems futile to work with a mentor who works outside your clinical field. It is precisely the prescribing relationship that permits authority and competency to progress. Therefore, work with doctors who have a close clinical association to your work.

As a nurse prescriber it is a fallacy to call yourself an independent prescriber. If you end up working independently, you may well end up working outside your clinical governance arrangements in your organisations. Nurse prescribing will work best when working as part of a team and in close collaboration with psychiatrists and other team members.

Be part of a network of nurse prescribers

Nurse prescribing is a global development and has succeeded well within the UK. Many innovative practices develop as nurse prescribers adapt and be adapted by the needs of the service. Learning from these experiences can be achieved by being part of local and national networks. National conferences organised by the Association of Nurse Prescribing are worthy networking opportunities.

Some organisations have set up newsletters that go out to all nurse prescribers outlining trust training days, medical and drug alerts and policy changes. A newsletter by itself garners support and sustains a collective feel to nurse prescribing. It helps to inform and keep nurses plugged into the live issues.

Build in support strategies

The journey of the nurse prescriber is long and arduous. Your managers and clinical advocates in the organisation need to believe that the implementation of nurse prescribing is worthwhile. Lots of energy is required to get through the hurdles of organisational anxiety. Helping your manager and psychiatrist in understanding the process of implementation will then help them to support you.

Some nurses believe, in error, that simply getting on the nurse prescribing course is the hardest hurdle. This is a misjudgement. Nurse prescribers need to cultivate and nurture their support mechanisms to ensure that the framework for practice is embedded into service design.

Understand the anxieties from medical staff and professions allied to medicine

There is a growth of nurse-prescribing activity but the frameworks are not universal across the UK. Many nurses and psychiatrists may feel that they are developing the process as implementation unfolds. This is an uncomfortable feeling for many clinicians. When nurse prescribing first started, NHS trusts developed the broad policy envelope to permit implementation. Some nurses may experience that different organisations have different levels of organisational anxiety about nurse prescribing. This may translate into unclear 'hoops' for nurses to jump through in order to prescribe.

To manage anxieties, nurses and doctors need to understand the roles of each professional group. Clarity about who manages the overall care package and the constituent parts of the care package is fundamental.

There need to be frequent discussion and reviews about the prescribing framework used by the nurse prescriber and the psychiatrist. Such reviews will not only inform the doctor about what is happening with the patient but also reduce anxieties if care and treatment are being delivered as planned.

The above sections are important because how other professions see the nursing profession and its drive to carry out a prescribing role will have an impact on its implementation. The nurse prescriber may wish to consider what expectations other professions have of the nurse prescriber and whether it is realistic. For example, by asking the question, the nurse prescribers may find that the psychiatrists believe the nurse prescribers will take away parts of their role or lead to changes in the job plan.

Get used to working to protocols and NICE guidelines

The direction of care within the NHS has been towards protocol-driven care. Nurses tend to adhere to protocols more than doctors. General practitioners express difficulty in using NICE guidelines in clinical practice (National Audit Office 2006). Protocols have been used successfully to guide the implementation of inpatient nurse prescribing (Harborne & Jones 2008). Protocols help nurses to stay within their limits of competency.

Protocols have also given way to more formalised evidence-based sets of standards within NICE guidance. Across mental health, they have been developed for all sorts of conditions and clinical situations (Box 4.1). They outline the accepted norms of diagnostic treatment for specified disorders.

Nurses can routinely adhere to NICE guidelines by including reference to them on their clinical management plans. Protocols governing the scope of prescribing competency can stipulate that nurses remain within the limits set down by guidelines. Protocols have many advantages, particularly in the defence of practice. A protocol demonstrates that senior clinicians have thought carefully

> **Box 4.1   Examples of guidance for mental health conditions.**
>
> Schizophrenia (NICE 2002a,b)   Bipolar disorder (NICE 2006c)
>
> Depression (NICE 2006b)   Insomnia (NICE 2004a)
>
> Smoking cessation (NICE 2006d)   Eating disorders (NICE 2004b)
>
> Dementia (NICE 2006a)   Disturbed and violent behav-
>   iour (NICE 2005a)

about the disease group and have considered the evidence supporting the intervention to be used. By doing this, it removes an element of risk where the nurse prescriber will obviously treat only those patients who they are familiar with. Uncertain, high-risk patients should be excluded from routine practice and their care and treatment overseen by psychiatrists.

Mental health nurses must bear in mind that they are the applicators of the protocols and guidance. In some situations, it may be inappropriate to follow the guidance or it may not best serve the patient at that particular moment in time. What is important is that the nurse has considered the guidance and has documented a clear decision-making trail, if this is different from the policy or guidance.

Clinical audit against protocol-driven care serves a useful way to determine what care has been given against agreed standards. Nurse-prescribing practice requires regular audit to ensure that parameters such as safety, prescribing patterns and satisfaction are reviewed. A successful audit process sustains implementation and further progresses, in this case prescriptive authority. Without a clear audit process, it can lead to senior 'culture carriers' to question the importance or value of nurse prescribing. Clinical audit therefore needs to become part of the culture of nurse prescribing.

Continuous professional development

The Nursing & Midwifery Council has determined that a minimum of 35h of learning activity over a 3-year period prior to registration is required for all nurses (Nursing & Midwifery Council 2008). Further to this, the Nursing & Midwifery Council (2008) is mindful that nurse prescribers are required to demonstrate revalidation of competency through more formal appraisal. A joint position statement by a range of health unions have put forward that continuous professional development should increase to 6 days of protected study time per year (Royal College of Nursing 2007). This stipulation would help on the nurse-prescribing development agenda. However, nurses must be clear on their own learning needs and how the organisation can help them to do this.

Following are the areas for nurses to consider for continuous professional development.

(1)　Assessment skills in history taking and mental state examination
(2)　Knowledge of mental health and coexisting medical conditions
(3)　Physical examination and impact on formulation and treatment
(4)　Psychopharmacology
(5)　Legal and professional policy issues

The overall goal of professional development is to bring about improved quality of care for patients, a lack of which may lead to adverse health outcomes (Nursing & Midwifery Council 2006). Concerns over nurse prescribing may be circumscribed by putting in place additional support and training. Nurse prescribers also need to receive feedback on the nurse-prescribing performance.

Nurse prescribers also need to think about how they can access both formal and informal methods of professional development. For example, some nurses like to receive information in a didactic fashion whilst others prefer an interactive approach. Nurses can ensure access to ongoing professional development through:

(1)　online learning through National Prescribing Centre, Association of Nurse Prescribing websites, and PRODIGY;
(2)　joining medical staff weekly sessions;
(3)　attending industry-sponsored meetings and conferences;
(4)　developing medication guidelines;
(5)　participating in video-recorded skills workshops;
(6)　having access to electronic journals and online support from medicines management websites;
(7)　undergoing direct supervision from their collaborating psychiatrist.

It is very easy for nurse prescribers to become preoccupied with their new prescriptive authority. Once they have taken the course and they are cognisant of their accountability framework, they see the patients regularly and maintain their records very well. Blind spots do emerge, which can be identified by exposing the nurse prescriber to a range of organisational and peer review monitoring systems. Outside speakers who are able to discuss their personal reflections on nurse prescribing in different areas help nurse prescribing to challenge the safety mechanisms that have been developed within the existing prescribing arrangements. They also help to facilitate a network arrangement so that arrangements do not become stale or unaffected by policy advances.

Medical practice has been subject to audit for over a decade. For nurse prescribing audit of prescriptions, conditions and outcomes not only help to reaffirm the safety of nurse prescribing but also add an element of transparency in terms of influence by the pharmaceutical companies. Forums of nurse prescribers can also consider more generalised information on the types of drugs that are being prescribed for conditions within the whole organisation. This will help to show whether there are any inconsistencies in the nurse-prescribing patterns.

Tensions with independent prescribing

Not all nurses, doctors and pharmacists who work in mental health agree that nurses should be an independent prescriber. They broadly think that independent prescribing is not safe for patients because nurses do not have the experience of clinical training that is available for medical staff.

However, what exactly is independent prescribing. It implies that the nurse enters the clinical problem as an independent practitioner and has the freedom to act as an independent practitioner. However, how can this be the case? Nurses work as part of a team, working side by side with other nurses, psychiatrists and general practitioners.

The concept of independent prescribing also brings up questions such as who owns the patient, or who is in charge of patient care. Traditionally, this is the general practitioner or the psychiatrist. They take on this responsibility by default or it is attributed to them. Consultant psychiatrists are responsible clin-icians under the Mental Health Act (2007). Why should they give up this responsibility? Independent prescribing assumes that the nurse will take on this authority for all aspects of patient care.

Another way of looking at independent prescribing is to think pragmatically about how care and treatment can be portioned out to relevant members of the care team. It may be that a patient has schizophrenia, diagnosed by a consultant and treatment prescribed appropriately. The patient enters into a crisis situation and starts to hear voices. A nurse prescriber may then prescribe a short-term sedative to reduce the arousal. In this sense, both the psychiatrist and the nurse prescriber have prescribed medication independently.

Transitions along the prescribing competency line

Organisations need to be clear how nurses are permitted to progress along to become an independent prescriber from a supplementary prescriber. Recent research demonstrates that nurses opt to work as a supplementary prescriber before taking on independent prescriptive authority (Kaplan & Brown 2007, Jones 2008). This could be because of confidence and an awareness to increase aspects of competency, which is perfectly understandable (Courtenay & Carey 2007). Nurses need to adapt to the new prescribing role and respond accordingly to the requirement for continuous professional development.

Develop a portfolio of cases

Development of a portfolio of cases should be where nurses demonstrates evidence of their prescribing activity. Nurses can describe the cases, key learning from their experience and reflections on where further sources of knowledge are required.

Prescribing activity should not be defined by the number of cases but by the amount of time spent in the area of prescribing activity. Some trusts have set the time as 1-year practice as a supplementary prescriber. The number of cases may be around 20, although there is no research exploring this issue.

Supervision and continuous professional development

In order for clinicians to progress to an independent prescriber, it is wise for an organisation to record the attendance at arranged training sessions on areas relevant for his or her prescribing practice.

Models of supervision for nurse prescribing are a developing area in terms of how nurses and doctors perceive this new form of relationship. Nurses are reliant on supervision for continued exchange of information and development of their competency parameters. Trusts assure clinicians of cover through vicarious liability on the grounds of continued supervision. Active engagement with the supervision process must be assured for nurses to progress to be an active independent prescriber.

Medical staff and their continued support for nurse prescribing are integral to its success. It is helpful for the nurses to meet with their supervisor on a monthly basis. It is important that the role of medical staff is thought through so that nurse prescribers can have a positive learning experience. Some reports from medical staff have identified the importance of clinical assessment skills to underpin nurse prescribing, which is the backbone in the latest guidance for independent prescribing (DoH 2006b). Doctors have a range of clinical experiences that help nurse prescribers during their mentorship phase. However, this comes with a requirement for time and financial compensation for the mentorship. Medical staff has also experienced problems where nurses tend to be much slower in their prescribing practice because they follow protocols. Doctors have also identified a diminishing trend in their role with the extension of nurse prescribing and the set of skills that sit alongside the prescribing role.

Nurse prescribing is a competency-based art that should be demonstrated continually in order for nurses to progress. It needs to be seen very much as nurses progressing through and accepting prescriptive authority depending on their level of knowledge, skill and competence.

There are issues as to how a psychiatrist is trained to assess the competency of the nurse prescriber. This requirement on the part of the psychiatrist is ongoing and may unearth a number of tensions. For example, the continuum of prescriptive authority suggests that competency can develop so that eventually it equals that of consultant psychiatrists in some areas of work.

Panels of experts

Some organisations have built in further safeguards to permit prescriptive authority to only those nurses who can demonstrate competency to experts in the field. A panel may consist of a medical and nursing director, chief pharmacists and a psychiatrist. The aspiring independent prescribing nurse then has to satisfy the requirements of this panel in order to gain prescriptive authority.

Medical delegation

It appears sensible for the independent prescribing nurses to have cases delegated to them from psychiatrists when they first start prescribing. It may appear that this is prescribing through a supplementary prescribing framework. However, there are clear differences. Even though the patient group may be selected, the independent prescriber will still be responsible for diagnosis or reconfirming diagnosis, starting treatment and then evaluating the treatment. The patients may not see the psychiatrist for a particular period during which the nurse prescriber is treating them. It seems difficult for independent prescribing to proceed unless organisations have a negotiated settlement over who will treat particular groups of patients.

Medical delegation can be further defined by spelling out circumstances where contact with a psychiatrist is required. Examples may be when the patient has uncommon symptoms or fails to progress along the treatment algorithm.

Competency

The key question to be addressed first is what precisely is competency.

For nurse prescribing, competency should be seen as a workplace activity. Progression to become an independent nurse prescriber will require higher levels of competency compared with a supplementary prescriber. The key question is not whether the persons themselves are competent but whether the activity they perform is competent. For example, the nurse may be competent to follow the process of being a nurse prescriber. But, would the nurse be competent in the titration of one drug to another? Competency in one area of prescribing practice would infer competency for other aspects (Nursing & Midwifery Council 2007).

Traditional methods of managing competency in medical and nursing circles are for clinicians to seek advice on how to proceed with an intervention before actually delivering it. The same must be adhered to for nurse prescribing. Nurses must see their work as being essentially distributed and delegated from medical staff. This may then help them to see that cases, depending on complexity, can shift back and forth along this line of competency. There should be no shame in observing and responding to your level of competency; indeed to do the opposite may put patients at risk of an untoward incident.

It is easy for clinicians to stray into areas closely associated with their main disease group but entirely different. An example would be of people with schizophrenia who develop comorbid hypercholesterolaemia and require a statin drug (drugs used to lower cholesterol). Unless the nurse prescriber undergoes separate training and this competency is assessed by his or her collaborating psychiatrist, he or she should resist such a temptation no matter how disruptive it may be to the patient to see another prescriber.

Nurse prescribing is a journey. Organisations need to think about how the journey can be mapped out so that there is some uniformity in determining competency across an agreed range of areas. Organisations can stipulate that nurses complete a learning log, which includes competency-based areas that need to be signed off by a responsible clinician who has assessed competency.

Areas that need to be included in the competency workbook mirror some already covered on the nurse-prescribing course. However, the difference here is the grounding of these skills in clinical practice using real-life prescribing practice.

As nurses demonstrate competency, their authority to prescribe can be extended. The situation becomes very much like a pilot, earning his or her wings with the number of flights he or she has piloted. The wings do not guarantee that the pilot will be able to manage all situations, but it does demonstrate sustained exposure to medically supervised practice and learning.

The concept of competency can be demonstrated for aspects of nurse-prescribing activity. The National Prescribing Centre (2003) has produced a set of competency statements in the form of a workbook; these competency statements are helpful in judging the level of competency for all nurse prescribers as they progress from simple titration to complex clinical management plans.

Organisations may wish to consider agreeing to a range of conditions that can be managed by a nurse prescriber. An example is of a nurse practitioner that has delegated responsibility to work with people who have depression, acute and chronic psychosis and mood disorder. The responsibility would be to initiate and switch treatment either in hospital or at home (if the patient is at home). The role and scope of the practitioner is agreed with the psychiatrist. This is not to say that all patients should have their care overseen by an independent prescriber. The assessment, diagnosis and management may best be overseen by the psychiatrist.

Progression of competency can be measured and reviewed annually. The psychiatrist is best placed to carry out this function. Tools to aid this would be to see if nurses have stayed within their scope of practice, review medication errors, report case notes, and issue external letters to general practitioners and other health professionals.

In order for nurse prescribers to carry on prescribing as a supplementary prescriber or to progress to an independent prescriber or retain this privilege, evidence of continued professional development should be collected over the past few years. If nurses are unable to do this, they should not be granted further prescriptive authority.

General principles of safe prescribing

Safe prescribing involves a number of different elements. An important area is to know your drugs and how the drugs work for particular conditions. This would mean prior experience in watching how the patient responds to the drug, observing for side effects and being knowledgeable about what is reasonable before carrying out the intervention. An example is the initiation of clozapine and how some patients with schizophrenia present with tachycardia after a few weeks of starting treatment of clozapine [drug licensed for the treatment of schizophrenia (BNF 2008)]. Nurses would continue to monitor this side effect but would consider repeating the electrocardiogram if the side effect continue beyond 3 months (Taylor *et al.* 2007).

Nurse prescribers need be able to navigate their way around the myriad of databases that contain the sources of evidence that support the treatment modality. In exceptional circumstances, nurse prescribers may carry out a search of the literature on drugs. For the most part, nurses should have available to them certain reference books that contain the evidence supporting certain treatments. For mental health, three textbooks are central to this process. The first is *The Maudsley Prescribing Guidelines* (Taylor *et al.* 2007). This book is on treatment algorithms, the chapters on side effects are revised annually and the book is key to safe prescribing practice. The second is Bazire's (2007) textbook on psychiatric drugs, again covering side effects but which gives quick and accessible information on drug contraindications. The third is Stahl's (2006) textbook, which helpfully gives 'easy-to-read' information on individual psychotropic drugs. Before prescribing medication, a nurse prescriber can have the most up-to-date information on how to prescribe the drug, how it works, how long it takes to work and what to do if it does not work. These ingredients underpin safe prescribing.

Quality of the patient record

The recording of clinical notes cannot be understated. More may be said by the nurse prescriber in the prescribing consultation than is documented in the clinical record. Nurse prescribing brings up a whole range of issues about the need for accurate details to be kept on why prescribing decisions have been made and what these prescribing decisions are and, if possible, also the evidence that supports the prescribing decision. The Nursing & Midwifery Council (2007) has produced guidelines for records. When nurse-prescribing decisions are made, they should be entered contemporaneously in the clinical record, as hard copy or in the electronic form, and the prescribing decision should be communicated to the immediate clinical team involved in the patient care. If this is not possible, arrangements need to be made where the clinical decision is accessible to the wider team.

The prescription itself must also be legible and correct. Surprisingly, one study found that significant differences existed between the quality of the written prescribing intervention for people with dementia (20% of prescriptions illegible) versus functional illness (anxiety and depression) (Nirodi & Mitchell 2002). Perhaps this indicates apathy towards the care of older people, but this needs to be reversed given the higher risks of untoward prescribing for this patient group.

Table 4.2   Golden rules about documentation for the nurse prescriber

Clarity of expression	Records are clear accounts for the patients care that are written legibly with limited use of abbreviations duly signed and dated.
Objective	The opinion of the nurse prescriber is based on what you know of the patients' history and mental state.
Contemporary	Notes are written at the time when the patient is being interviewed or soon after the interview has been completed.
First hand	The nurse prescriber actually writes their own notes as opposed to another clinician.
Tamper-proof	The entry is written in pen and any spaces are scored through.
Sufficient detail	The frequency and detail of note keeping may need to increase if patients are deemed to be complex and require more intensive contact than normal.

Case law will require the defence to demonstrate adequate record keeping for the intervention carried out. One way for nurses to understand this dilemma is to imagine that their records are being used in their defence. It is important for them to realise that if their actions have not been written down, they have not been completed. The point about record keeping is that it should demonstrate that you have understood and delivered your duty of care and that actions and omissions on the part of the nurse prescriber have not compromised patient safety. The quality of records can be improved by nurses considering the headings given in Table 4.2.

Dealing with drug errors

Nurses will make drug errors in their prescribing practice just like doctors and dentists have always done. It is inevitable because any human activity is prone to mistakes. Drug errors lead to increased hospital admission time and cause harm and risk to patients' lives (DoH 2004b). Even when nurses commit these errors, they can be traumatic for the individual. What is unknown as yet is how a nurse prescriber will react to committing a drug error and what impact this will have on his or her prescribing practice.

Medication errors occur at all stages of prescription. They can never be eliminated, but a system can be designed that makes it difficult for the nurse prescriber to make a mistake (Reason 1990). When medication errors occur, it is usually a systems failure or a combined multidisciplinary team failure (O'Shea 1999) as opposed to a reckless act on the part of the prescriber.

Medication errors are an indicator of quality used to demonstrate patient safety (DoH 2004b). The majority of medication errors result in no harm to the patient, although the direct costs are up to 400 million per annum (DoH 2004b). Medication errors occur substantially (up to 70%) when patients are admitted into hospitals. Systems can be designed to minimise this risk by checking

Table 4.3   Causes of drug errors commonly seen in clinical practice

Drug dose, frequency and administration	Poor medication history taking on admission
Similar-sounding names of drugs	Lack of knowledge
Use of abbreviations	Non-adherence to policy
Complicated drug regimens	Busy routine
Patients taking the wrong medication	Poor communication between the prescriber and the patient at the time of prescription and failure to check understanding

that the drug history before admission matches that upon admission (National Prescribing Centre 2008). Medication errors result in delayed discharge from hospital of up to 8 days (Vincent *et al.* 2001).

When one looks at medication errors, two types emerge, the first being lapses of concentration and the second, a more serious one, being lack of knowledge (Dean *et al.* 2002). Many factors contribute to prescribing errors and the most common are included in Table 4.3 (Leape *et al.* 1995; DoH 2004b). Nurse prescribers, being more informed about drugs, may reduce drug errors from occurring.

Reporting concerns about medication

Nurse prescribers need to consider what type of product they are wishing to prescribe; particularly for mental health, safety issues should be paramount. Nurse prescribers need to have not only skills in the detection of the common adverse drug reactions associated with the drug but also awareness of less common examples. This requires an open mind when patients present to them with adverse drug reactions that are not commonly seen in clinical practice.

The Medicines & Healthcare Products Regulatory Agency (MHRA) operates a system where nurse prescribers complete the 'Yellow Card' found in the back of the British National Formulary (BNF 2008). Nurses are good at reporting concerns about side effects of medication via this mechanism. Patients themselves may prefer to report their own concerns. The onus is on the nurse prescriber to make sure the patient is aware of the procedure.

Prescribing for patients you have not seen

There are two occasions when this may occur. The first occasion is when it is easy to fall into a position where you may take information from another clinician in the team and make a prescribing decision. This occurs frequently in primary care but this practice should not be replicated by nurse prescribing. The whole purpose of nurse prescribing is to improve on medical prescribing.

The second occasion is more serious. This is where nurse prescribers, more likely to be independent prescribers, may prescribe medication for patients they have not assessed. The example will be the patient who has come into hospital in acute distress. Information will be relayed to the nurse prescriber from other nurses in the team. The nurse prescriber may then act on this advice and prescribe medication. This is poor prescribing practice and does nothing to enhance compliance or satisfy concerns over patient safety.

Renewal of prescriptions

It is commonplace for medication charts to be rewritten or for drugs to be prescribed from the original list. It is also commonplace for *de facto* prescribing to take place where the nurse would copy out the list of prescriptions and then take a doctor's signature on the form. This often happens in primary care. It seems much better for the nurse prescriber to be allowed to write a renewal prescription for drugs. However, underlying this practice change should be a list of drugs that the nurse prescriber is not allowed to renew unless he or she works in the particular area. An example would be of a nurse working in substance misuse who is familiar with the use of methadone for heroin addiction to renew the prescription.

Separate out prescribing from dispensing

The prescribing of medication is different from the dispensing of medication. Dispensing medication is where the nurse gives out medication from a treatment plan. Clinical governance dictates that all organisations have a policy to ensure safe dispensing of medication. Nurse prescribers must guard against situations where they prescribe medication and then dispense it. It may occur in emergency situations. The nurse prescriber prescribes intramuscular haloperidol for rapid tranquilisation and then ends up administering it as part of a treatment team [drug licensed for the treatment of short-term treatment of agitation (BNF 2008)]. Nurse prescribers may end up mixing the two responsibilities if they are involved in the clinical situation. The basic rule is not to mix prescribing and dispensing no matter how innocuous the situation looks when it first appears.

Stay within the management plan or formulary guidelines

For nurses who work with a clinical management plan, medicines or groups of medicines are agreed with the psychiatrists. It is important for nurse prescribers to stay within the parameters of what they have agreed with the psychiatrist. The British National Formulary is revised twice a year and it is a key reference for nurse prescribers. The British National Formulary offers guidance on what the drug is licensed to do and the dose ranges. It is for general guidance, and unless nurses are particularly experienced in their field of practice, they would be advised to stay within them.

Nurses who are experienced in the treatment of particular disorders and in the use of defined types of medication may feel comfortable operating outside British National Formulary guidance. However, nurses should always be able to reference back their prescribing decision to evidence, case study research and, at best, protocols. If nurses do depart from British National Formulary guidelines, they will be expected to defend their decisions in the event of untoward incidents.

It is important that nurse prescribers prescribe medication that is indicated for the condition at a dose that is effective, and that this information is documented clearly both in the prescription itself and in the prescription card, if in hospital settings, and in the notes.

Conclusion

The reality of nurse prescribing is that it is in early days of implementation. Models of implementation have been explored where nurses are taking the lead in managing patient groups across the care pathway. Ways of overcoming organisational and professional inertia and negative viewpoints have been discussed. Key to bringing about implementation is to share best practice and success stories. Research studies are helpful but more mileage may be found by championing local policies, case studies and conference reports.

To address implementation deficit, the first most important message would be for trusts and employing organisations to search out which areas of the service would benefit from a nurse prescriber most. The second message would be to look at the area of the service where nurse prescribing is most successful. Wrapped up with successful nurse prescribing is a robust clinical governance structure within healthcare organisations. General principles of good prescribing have been reviewed that support patient safety.

The importance of nurses to practice safely within their competency has also been reviewed. The progression to become an independent prescriber requires careful assessment in terms of competency but also how it would meet the needs of the organisation.

Chapter 5
History and assessment: The basis for effective nurse prescribing

Introduction

This chapter is split into three sections. Section 1 will take the reader through the process of recording a history. In order to provide some form to this chapter, the process of taking a history for working-age adults will be discussed. A few important texts that are recommended to be read alongside this chapter include the early works of Wing *et al.* (1974), who set out the present state examination, and Gelder *et al.* (2004), who listed the major headings for taking a history and mental state. Poole & Higgo (2006) provided a contemporary understanding of the process that is again useful for the nurse prescriber.

Section 2 will outline the process of carrying out a mental state examination, which usually takes place at the time of interview. Ideally, the mental state examination should follow on from the history-taking process. The process is applicable to old-age, adult and substance misuse areas. Each area within this broad church approaches the patient wanting to know different aspects of medical history and symptom presentation. The assessment identified here majors on adult services, as more specialist areas of assessment would be required for particular presentations.

Section 3 will cover the process of carrying out a consultation and arriving at a diagnosis and formulation. The process of nurse prescribing is not just about giving medication to patients. In fact, the prescribing of medication occurs at the end of an assessment process and, for many patients, will not even happen at all. It is important to arrive at an assessment and formulation that helps clinicians and patients to understand what is happening.

Section 1: Why is history important?

The process of taking a history enables the prescriber to understand how the patient's symptoms are presenting. The assessment will inform the prescriber whether a disorder is present and to what degree, how long symptoms have been present and what is the effect those symptoms have on the patient's life.

What is the process?

Standardised ways of taking a history were described by Gelder *et al.* (2004). There are positive aspects to this process, given that it can be rehearsed so that the clinician becomes proficient in assessing and collecting information. Other clinicians familiar with the psychiatric history can also follow the history, test the hypothesis and gather further information from subsequent interviews.

What do you intend to find out?

The psychiatric history is taken under a series of commonly used headings (Box 5.1). All of the sections are important to complete a history and pertinent sections are discussed in further detail. For nurse prescribers who are not familiar with the process, it may be helpful to make note of the headings and then to use them to structure your interview.

Box 5.1   Components to the history taking process.

- Biographical details
- History of presenting condition
- Family history
- Personal history
- Past medical conditions
- Personality function
- Use of illicit substances, alcohol, nicotine

Presenting complaint and history of the presenting complaint

This category is the first section to a history. A question revolves around what has brought patients into contact with psychiatric services or for review at follow-up. You may recall some psychiatrists typically ask patients 'why have you come to see me today', even though it was a prearranged outpatient appointment. For patients who newly present to the service or have altered symptom presentation, it is a really important stage to record how they made contact, which professional saw them and what symptoms they presented with. Nurse prescribers must differentiate between symptoms that are present at the time of interview and those that are part of the history of the presenting complaint.

Most emergency assessments are highly charged and it is important to record this because, undoubtedly, when the situation becomes controlled, this will be lessened. An example is a 19-year-old man who recently broke up with his girlfriend and then impulsively takes an overdose and, in the process, throws himself in front of the police car. The furore surrounding the presenting complaint should be distinguished from the presenting mental state.

When this section of the history is scant, the nurse prescriber (if not the admitting nurse) may have to assume that the symptoms they presented with were the same as what you see in later interviews. An example is a patient who presents to an accident and emergency department with ideas that people are spreading rumours that he or she is a paedophile and shows symptoms of arousal, disturbed sleep and disorganised thinking. The patient is then admitted to the ward and given a mild sedative to control arousal. With the calm environment of the ward, sleep hygiene and a sedative, the arousal diminishes, and the following day, the assessing clinician is left with a presentation of vague ideation that people may be talking about the patient, but the patient does not know why. A clearly described history of the presenting complaint gives the subsequent psychiatric interview a context to probe further. This is why you need to record a history of each symptom, when it started and for how long it has been present.

The nurse prescriber should allow the patient to go into more depth about the events leading to the assessment, or the admission. The presentation sets the context for the assessment. The interview must be allowed to proceed at the pace set by the patient and to let the story unfold. The interviewer can seek clarification on various points by paraphrasing, questioning and comparing the 'present' with the 'past'.

Personal history

This is a large compilation of factors that need to be considered. Sections to the personal history should cover birth, relationships, schools, employment, and personal relationships. This allows the nurse to build a pen picture of the patient. Not all areas will be covered in sufficient depth at the first interview but these can be added iteratively as the interview and the process of assessment and formulation continue.

A useful place to start is to consider the birth and the subsequent development of the child, through schooling and scholastic achievement. The interviewer may prompt patients to consider any difficulties with their birth and whether they reached milestones such as walking and talking. The interviewer may discover past difficulties at school, such as bullying or truanting. You may want to start the process by asking the patients to talk about their childhood or to recall important memories, good and unpleasant. The aim of these questions is to encourage them to tell their personal stories. However, questions need to be purposeful as an overinclusive personal history may distract attention from the task of eventual formulation.

The interviewer may discover that the patient achieved well at school, passing exams to enter a university to study law. The nurse may unearth early symptoms suggestive of a depressive disorder when the patient was in his second year. For example, the patient may have isolated himself and lost interest in study, resulting in poor educational achievement when he left the university. In other words, a change has occurred from the expected trajectory.

It is also important to ask patients about their employment history – when they started working, how long they stayed in work, reasons for leaving and job attainment. The interviewer may find that the patients are unable to sustain long periods of employment and it would be helpful to ask them why this happens. They may identify socially acceptable reasons for leaving employment. Careful questioning may reveal whether the poor employment record was part of a trajectory or indeed a marker for social withdrawal and a developing mental illness.

A genogram helps to illustrate patients' relationships with their parents and siblings. The role that children play within the family often follows them into adulthood and gives a viewpoint on their esteem and position within the family. The psychiatric history places a great deal of value on the family context. The genogram places the patient within a context, for example, whether the patient is the youngest of five siblings. It is important to identify the age of the parents, their jobs, any medical conditions they may suffer, whether they are deceased and, if so, the cause of death. From the genogram, the nurse could focus on any difficulties in the family, parent–child relationships or tensions. The interviewer may find out that the mother spent frequent and prolonged periods of time during the day in the pub. One could draw conclusions about the influence of parental nurture and love during children's developmental years. It is important to ask patients about their interpretation to family events and to hold at bay your own cultural norms.

In this section, you may discover that the patient's father was diagnosed with a depressive disorder, resulting in hospital admission. A genetic predisposition could then be considered when identifying possible reasons for the presenting complaint. The family history may also reveal that, in the past, family members attempted or committed suicide. This genetic link is important for predicting further risks for the patient.

The family history should contain pointers to the patient's upbringing. Some patients may come from separated parents and go on to describe the dynamics of living with a single parent. The personal history should include who the patient lives with and if he or she has dependent children. Another important question here is: who has parental responsibility for the dependent child? It is important to have this issue clarified at interview. Evidence suggests that children of parents with a mental illness also carry a risk of developing mental illness (Rutter & Quinton 1984) and so the needs of the children should also be considered. The assessing nurse has a responsibility to assess any child protection and safe guarding issues.

The personal history should also contain information about patients' current social context, where they are living and who they are living with. They may say that they are presently single and live in a one-bedroom council flat. They may disclose that they have little or no support from their family and friends. Again the personal history begins to point towards a risk formulation that will guide the current management plan.

Sexual history is important and can be covered in this section. This could be addressed by asking patients when they had their first sexual experience and if this was with same sex or opposite sex. The aim of the questions is not to pry into their private life but to determine if sexual disturbance has led or contributed to the presenting complaint. The nature and delivery of the questions need to be sensitive and purposeful. On a more practicable level, there are examples of psychotropic medication such as selective serotonin reuptake inhibitors prescribed for depression that cause sexual dysfunction (BNF 2008) and these problems can be identified at the psychiatric interview.

Financial history

In today's society, many people are burdened by debt or suffer financial worries that cause or worsen mental distress. Financial difficulties may actually be a symptom of mania such as overspending because of grandiose ideation and poor impulse control. The interviewer should ask patients about their present debt and difficulties of living with this.

Past medical history

It is unlikely that nurses will have at their command the range of knowledge about the various diseases that affect the body. Ask patients open questions about their health and illness. An inventory of minor illness and diseases is not required. However, the clinician should record major diseases that resulted in serious physical, psychological and social traumas. Issues to note would be infections like encephalitis or major fractures or medical conditions. Major surgical operations should also be noted with dates. A note needs to be made whether the surgery was related to particular traumas through accidents or self-injurious behaviours.

Nurse prescribers need to consider the age of individuals and the likelihood of developing medical conditions. Some people may develop diseases of ageing far quicker than usual and this should be noted. The natural process of ageing would also lead to medical conditions such as cardiovascular disease and diabetes. Chapter 6 discusses a range of infectious, neurological and metabolic disorders that coexist with mental illness. Careful recording of these conditions, treatment and likely impact on prospective psychiatric treatment is required. For example, it would be unwise to prescribe olanzapine [drug licensed for the treatment of schizophrenia (BNF 2008)] to a patient who was obese and had type 2 diabetes. Lithium for bipolar affective disorder would be contraindicated in patients with an impaired renal system (BNF 2008).

Past psychiatric history

In this section, the nurse would make a note of what conditions the patients have been diagnosed with and whether they received ongoing treatment. In essence, you need to know if the patients are currently known to psychiatric services or if they have been treated by services in a different part of the country. It would be insufficient to record 'known to psychiatric services' because the splitting of modern-day services into different types of teams provides an indication of the severity of illness. A patient who is managed by the assertive outreach team is likely to have a protracted illness trajectory and carry a significant amount of risk of poor engagement. It would be useful to look back on past episodes of accident and emergency contact and how the presenting complaint was managed. If the patient had presented with past attempts to self-harm, the interviewer must record whether the patient was admitted to hospital and whether the attempt of self-harm reached lethal levels. The trigger to the self-harm event would be noted and considered against frequency and intensity. The interviewer should record dates and outcomes for each event, such as receiving medical intervention and any subsequent mental health assessment. The interviewer would want to arrive at a view on whether there is an escalation of self-harm attempts over time or if it is part of a usual pattern of behaviour.

Episodes of inpatient hospital treatment must be noted, along with reasons for admission, treatment, duration of stay and date of admission – importantly, whether the person has ever been admitted to hospital under the Mental Health Act and there is any noted risk to self or others. If the patient had previously been admitted to hospital, it is important to make a note of the care coordinators and which mental health team they are based in. The important point is to make a note of the outcome of treatment and what worked and what failed.

Medication history

There are three sections to a medication history. The first relates to the taking of alcohol, caffeine and nicotine and illicit drug misuse. An alcohol history would include the amount of alcohol consumed each week, differentiating between drinks having low and high alcohol content, and the time of consumption; for example, a heavy binge-drinking episode every 2 weeks may be problematic and lead to social disruption and criminal activity. Others are habitual and drink alcohol daily. The history would include the amounts of alcohol per day, which will total to a weekly amount.

Caffeine is a drug that leads to heightened sense of arousal and anxiety when taken in excess. Many everyday products contain caffeine (see Chapter 6) and a drug history would include the types of drinks and when they are taken. For example, patients on clozapine [drug licensed for the treatment of schizophrenia (BNF 2008)] may consume two to three cups of coffee to give them the stimulus to break through the morning sedation. Alternatively, the drug history may reveal that a patient drinks coffee in the late hours of the evening, which disturbs the sleep cycle.

Illicit drug misuse is a commonly occurring habit that requires careful assessment. People self-medicate using cannabis to promote relaxation or amphetamines to give themselves a feeling of euphoria, which may be referred to as a 'buz'. Charting substance misuse gives an indication of the patient's social lifestyle and whether the patient has underlying addictive personality traits. People also misuse legal drugs. For example, procyclidine [drug used to treat extrapyramidal side effects (BNF 2008)] can be taken as a stimulant. Patients may sell or give away medication to others, so asking about this adds to the overall formulation.

The second section includes drugs that have been prescribed previously and currently, certainly for mental illness and other medical conditions. If accessible, information can be obtained from the general practitioner records by contacting the surgery. Polydrug misuse needs to be kept in mind, so checking with patients if they are registered with different general practitioners is important. There are occasions when people are admitted to hospital and report that they are in receipt of methadone and give false information on the dose or frequency of administration. In these circumstances, the nurse prescriber would refrain from prescribing these drugs until verification has taken place.

Nurse prescribers also need to keep in mind that people buy over-the-counter medication such as pain killers, herbal anxiolytics and St John's wort for depression. Antidepressant medication, for example, should not be prescribed if the patient is also taking St John's wort (BNF 2008). Certain over-the-counter medications such as paracetamol also carry drug allergies that patients may not identify as such and may also interact with the drug prescribed. The interviewer must ascertain if the patients had benefited from previously prescribed drugs and for how long they have been taking the drugs.

A medication history should be taken with the patient but also separately by going through the patient notes. General advice is to start with a time line and to identify when the patient started taking the drug, including its dose and dose changes, and when he or she stopped taking it. Reasons for stopping the drug should also be noted if recorded. Equally, a positive response to the drug should also be recorded, as quite often, drugs change with little consideration. The time line should record all psychotropic drugs. Along with this time line, it is also useful to record the diagnosis and whether this changes over time or if the patient has a cluster of conditions.

The third section relates to known patient allergies to medication. This is important to note before nurses take the decision to prescribe an injection formulation. Some patients may have a previous reaction to medication, so prescribing it again without checking would be a drug error.

Forensic history

The patient may not be forthcoming with items of forensic history. It is important to ask about spent and current convictions. Periods of arrest, bail, probation and prison detention are important to note. Some patients receive a mental health assessment whilst being detained in prison or held on remand. These assessments provide important clues to their future risk and whether mental illness has any bearing on offending behaviour.

Prompts to aid this part of the history are to ask the patient about past episodes of being drunk and disorderly and whether the patient was arrested and subsequently convicted. People may become less controlled over their behaviour when they are drunk.

The interviewer should take a record of all spent convictions and what custodial and noncustodial actions were taken. This is important because some patients may try to feign mental illness in order to be diverted from the criminal justice system.

Premorbid functioning as a teenager should be recorded, including whether the patient truanted and engaged in antisocial behaviour. Questions to prompt this may be to ask the patient if he or she engaged in dangerous or exciting behaviours and any subsequent actions.

An index offence is where the patient has been arrested and convicted for carrying out a criminal act whilst being mentally unwell. The forensic history would record the circumstances leading to the index offence and any subsequent admission to environments of low, medium or high security.

Premorbid personality

This aspect is approached by asking patients what they were like before they became ill or unwell with their psychiatric problems. Of course, some people may not view their problems as being 'psychiatric'. Patients can be prompted to give a description of their character, habits and attitudes towards life or people; their relationships with family, friends and work colleagues; and how they spend their time in leisure and the types of leisure pursuits.

Lastly, it is important to collect a description on patients' predominant mood when they go about daily life. Here, a further prompt may be to suggest to the patient how other people would describe them. Patients can also be asked to mention their strengths and weaknesses and to describe their usual coping strategies. For example, some people may cope with excess pressure at work by taking recreational drugs at the weekend. Others may use alcohol every night. A more structured assessment of personality disorder may be the Structured Clinical Interview for DSM-IV Axis II Personality Disorders SKID 2 (First *et al.* 1997). This is useful for giving an informed view on personality types such as schizoid, avoidant and dependent personality traits. The interview is carried out when the patients are in a stable phase and when the interviewer has built a rapport and is able to triangulate the information given by them.

Issues for older people

The process outlined above is largely similar to that for older people. There is a greater tendency to develop disorders like heart disease, diabetes and respiratory disorders in old age. Thyroid disorders also mimic mental disorders. Nurse prescribers also need to be aware that younger adults and people with learning disability can develop organic conditions.

Substance misuse is common in older people and frequently misdiagnosed. Older people may place less emphasis on only taking medication prescribed for them. They may borrow medication from family or friends in the common belief that general types of medication are the same. Older people may take their medication for periods longer than necessary, at doses higher than prescribed or along with alcohol (Gossop & Moos 2008). The effects of medication on older people are particularly troublesome and causative to cognitive impairment that mimics dementia.

Issues for co-occurring learning disability

People with learning disability may be difficult to interview. They may have difficulties in understanding the questions put to them or difficulty in expressing themselves. They may also present with a host of medical disorders that commonly coexist, such as epilepsy.

Aspects of the personal history are relevant to pregnancy and birth. Difficulties with the development of the foetus or difficulties in birth resulting in brain damage need to be recorded. Patients with learning disability may not pass through the usual developmental milestones, so this needs to be considered. Childhood diseases and viral diseases may also have resulted in disability.

Issues for substance misuse

Patients who present with a clear-cut substance misuse disorder will require a detailed history to consider coexisting medical disorders and mental health. We know that people often take more alcohol than what they think or what they reveal, so any alcohol history must be seen as a conservative estimate. A particular concern for people who misuse substances is the level of depression and poor physical health that they suffer (Harvard *et al.* 2006).

A full alcohol history should include how much alcohol is taken, for how long it has been taken and what is its impact on life. A trigger question would be to ask about the patient's occupational history. People with alcohol problems may start off with an aspiring career but experience decline as the effects of alcohol misuse take its toll on maintaining employment stability, given sickness, unreliability, use of alcohol at work and work incompetence. The impact of sustained alcohol misuse would also have an impact on family and friends. A trigger question may be to ask if any family or friends have commented on their alcohol consumption and, if they have, what areas of their lifestyle have changed.

Alcohol increases the morbidity and mortality risk from breast, cervix, mouth, stomach and liver cancers (Gilmore & Sheron 2007; World Cancer Research Fund 2007). Careful examination of alcohol-related conditions when taking the past and current medical history is important. Some patients may not link their alcohol consumption to a medical problem.

Substance misuse history taking must not be limited to working-age people. The history-taking process must take account of the fact that people of older age consume alcohol in excess of agreed limits and that substance misuse worsens coexisting medical conditions that go hand in hand with the ageing process (Moos *et al.* 2004).

Issues for adult areas

The most important point is gender. The nurse should ask patients if they are pregnant and how they would confirm this. If they are, nurse prescribers need to flag up issues about breastfeeding and the choice of medication that can be offered. Nurse prescribers must ask all women if they have conceived or are planning to conceive. Some medication is tetragenic, meaning that it causes irreversible foetal changes. Some drugs such as valproate should not be prescribed to women of child-bearing age (Taylor *et al.* 2007).

Issues for all areas

The process of taking a history takes time to perfect. Nurse prescribers need to learn the art and craft of interviewing and then recording information at the same time. The history-taking process should take into account the emotional context that people find themselves in. Patients should be informed that you are a nurse, and with their permission, you would like to collect this information as part of your assessment as a nurse prescriber.

Some patients may not be able to give information pertaining to their history or symptoms, so collecting information from relatives, carers and friends is of importance. Where the interviewer finds that the patient lacks capacity as a result of the history-taking process, this should be flagged up and procedures followed for this eventuality. One of the guiding principles is that patients have the capacity to take their own decisions unless the nurse prescriber thinks otherwise. Nurse prescribers should continually seek to explain the treatment and to check that the patient understands the information. One strategy that can be recorded is advanced treatment directives, where patients are asked to state what they would like to be done if they lose the capacity to take decisions (DoH 2008a). An example is people who, when they relapse, require rapid tranquilisation with psychotropic medication.

Health professionals need to be aware of the stigma attached to being mentally ill and using illicit substances. Such prejudice may prevent these groups from seeking treatment for physical and mental health problems (DoH 2006d; Rethink 2006), thus worsening their outcome. A large study has shown that people who are addicted to alcohol or drugs are the most stigmatised group (Crisp *et al.* 2005) and the same can be said for people who suffer from a personality disorder (Thornicroft 2006).

People who are drug addicted and who may be more at risk of blood-borne viruses such as HIV cannot be seen as any less worthy of treatment. This calls for nurse prescribers, as well as all health professionals, to hold at bay their prejudiced views on treating people who may be HIV infected. Discriminatory views may be so toxic as to exclude such people from treatment (Mason *et al.* 2001); therefore, cultural understanding on the part of the nurse prescriber is required.

Fundamental to the history-taking process is good communication skills. When talking to patients, the nurse prescriber needs to refrain from using jargon-laden language to gather information. When information is received, the nurse should record it in a nonjudgemental way and not comment on the consultation.

Section 2: Why do a mental state examination?

The mental status examination is a process that can be learnt. Similar to the process of taking a history, there is a process for taking a mental state. It is taught to medical students as part of their training. Nurse prescribers would also have been tested on the ability and knowledge to undertake a mental state examination as part of their prescribing course requirements. The process of taking a history gives many clues to the mental state, but it is important to remember the distinction between the two processes.

What is the process?

The main components to a mental state examination are:

- appearance and behaviour;
- speech and mood;
- delusions and perceptual disturbance;
- orientation and cognition;
- insight.

Appearance and behaviour

The aim of this section is to give a description of how patients look like when they present to an interview. The way they dress and their self-care say a lot about their mental state. The examination is to note whether the patient is groomed or dishevelled, that is, the state and quality of the clothing. The odour of patients may indicate the level of self-care. It may indicate metabolic disorders (diabetes) if the smell of ketones is noted. It is also important to note patients' facial expressions, level of eye contact and whether their heads are bowed. Also recorded is the way patients enter the examination room and their behaviour through the examination process. For example, the patient may be agitated, restless or anxious. The extent to which the patient can sustain the interview process is also noted. Patients may start off being calm and collected, but at the end, they may be wringing their hands. Some patients who present with sullen mood may bear scars of past episodes of self-harm. It would be useful to record them if they are visible on the patient's arms or wrists.

The patient's overall behaviour should be recorded. For example, patients may enter the room in an animated fashion, as though they had special powers such as combat training and are overly familiar with battle routines. They may display an abnormal posture by holding their body in an odd position. Quite often, patients may show repeated and regular movements that are not goal directed. Some patients may present with a symptom called 'echopraxia', where they copy the movement of the examiner or another person in the room.

Manner

The examiner should note whether the patient is hostile towards the interview process or helpful with answering questions. A patient who has taken amphetamines may be irritable and abuse the clinician by calling his or her name or being provocative. A patient who is depressed may be solemn during the interview process.

It is important to note how patients engage in the interview, whether they are slumped into the chair or lying around on the settee at home or falling on the floor in the ward environment. They may be overactive or have retarded movements. These should be noted as part of the interview process.

Appropriateness

The pertinent question to consider here is whether patients are in 'touch' with their surroundings. You may want to observe if the patient is distracted by stimuli that are noticed by the interviewer or that are only experienced by the patient.

Mood and affect

Questions relating to mood should not be confused with simply finding out if the patient is depressed one day and fine the next day. One way to do this is to differentiate between mood and affect. Affect is how the patient expresses his or her emotion at the time of interview. For example, does the patient have a blunted or flat affect? A blunted affect is where the patient may not be able to express a full emotional response to a situation. A flat affect is where there is no emotion expressed.

Mood is emotion that prevails over a period of time. For example, the patient may report feeling low over the last 2 weeks. Mood symptoms cross all types of functional and organic conditions. The important point is to accurately assess mood symptoms and then to consider the symptoms within a particular diagnostic classification.

It is important to ask patients how they report their mood and this is called a subjective impression. They can be asked about their energy levels and motivation to initiate and sustain everyday life activities. Patients may report difficulties in 'getting going' in the mornings or their mood deteriorating or improving as the day progresses. They can also be asked about their libido and whether they have a healthy sexual response.

Patients may not express a sad mood but may be worried about life events or have excessive guilt about concerns, over and above usual mood. A differentiating question here is to ask patients to describe how they have been feeling over the last 2 weeks. Patients can be asked about their plans for the future. They may say they feel depressed and suicidal but then go on to talk about a planned holiday with friends. The point to be made here is whether the patient has mood congruence. Patients can be asked about their feelings of hopelessness. People who feel hopeless may express this as 'doesn't matter what happens, nothing will change'. Patients who feel helpless or worthless may again report that they have no control over events to become better.

For patients with a psychotic disorder, their mood may be incongruous to the situation. Patients may express contentment or appear 'nonplussed' when remembering the death of a loved relative. Mood in this sense may appear blunted.

The mental state record must include whether the patients have any suicidal thoughts, whether they have made any plans, what their means of committing suicide would be and what their intent is. Contrary to misconception, asking patients about their suicidal thoughts does not increase suicidal ideation or acts (NICE 2006b).

It is important for the examiner to distinguish between suicide-related behaviour and suicidal ideation. The former is an all-round term that describes all self-inflicted behaviours such as taking pills and laceration where the intention was not to kill themselves. Ideation suggests that intentional self-harm behaviours may occur in the future. It is a skilled task to elicit these responses and to separate out the behaviour that gives the impression that patients want to end their life when, in fact, they do not wish to die.

People who abuse substances may also complain of low mood and having suicidal thoughts with evidence of guilt and low self-esteem. They may have low mood, ruminating on the consequences of their self-destructive behaviour. Separating out alcohol-induced mood disorder from an underlying depressive disorder can be difficult.

Thoughts

What goes through people's minds is the subject of intense scrutiny in a mental state examination. Careful recording of the speech is vital in terms of the content, flow and form of thoughts. Nurses need to record pertinent sentences that reflect pathological thought content.

The interviewer may want to note whether the patient has any abnormal thought content that reaches a delusional intensity or whether the thoughts are one of an overvalued idea. Delusions can be mood congruent or mood incongruent. Delusions can follow particular themes such as being persecuted, grandiose or paranoid. An example is a patient who believes the neighbours are recording his or her conversations. The patient has a strongly held conviction that is not amenable to an alternative explanation.

You may wish to ask patients about who has control over their thoughts. A trigger question here is: do you have control over your thoughts? Patients may believe that thoughts are being implanted into their brains to carry out actions and instructions being sent from a computer in the community centre. The element to be distinguished here is passivity phenomena and if the patients think they have control over their thoughts or thoughts are being controlled from an external source.

The interviewer should elicit if there is thought broadcasting, by asking the patient if people know what he or she is thinking. You will need to prompt the patient to explain how this occurs. For example, the patient may report that people in the town centre can receive 'brain messages' about their movements in hospital. Citizens then respond to this by purposefully ignoring them (this would be a usual response if there is no past acquaintance) and the patients interpret this as a shun because they are thinking 'bad thoughts'.

Patients may have reduced thought content. This may be examined by asking the patients to respond to a range of questions about how they are and what they plan to do. They may be unable to give any detail or content to what they think.

Patients may also express thoughts that go from one subject to another, otherwise known as flight of ideas. They may appear incoherent and difficult to follow. The form of thoughts may appear disjointed and have unclear links, otherwise known as loosening of association. This should not be confused with 'knights move thinking', where the patient jumps from one topic to another but there is no logical sequence. The most extreme form of thought disorder is word salad, where conversations cannot be understood.

Depressed patients may express negative thoughts about the past, the present and the future. Trigger questions here would be whether the patients see themselves as hopeless, helpless or guilt ridden because of past or imaginary misdemeanours. They may express overvalued ideas about past events and make out that a situation or event has profound implications for their life events.

Some patients may have irrational obsessive thoughts. They may recognise these but are unable to resist the intrusive nature of them. Patients may have irrational thoughts about being dirty or being near dirty objects or may fear being contaminated by travelling on the train. If patients express these thoughts, the follow-on question is to ask about their ritualistic behaviours. For example, some patients may wash their hands five times, thinking about being dirty.

Perceptions

Patients may experience stimuli not experienced by the assessing clinician. Patients may hear noises, sounds or voices inside their head or outside their head, in the room or outside the room. The voices may be talking to the patient (second person) about the patient or talking to another person about the patient (third person). Hallucinations can also affect the sense of taste, smell or touch. Patients who are withdrawing from alcohol may experience tactile hallucinations and describe an itching sensation. Visual hallucinations can also occur in this circumstance and the most frequent sensory disturbance is seeing spiders in the room.

Patients may complain about hearing voices, but they may express this as their own thoughts. The interviewer should elicit whether what is being experienced is their own voice inside their head or whether the voice originates outside their head but within the room or outside the room. A trigger question here is to ask patients whether they think other people can hear their thoughts being spoken out aloud.

As part of the interview process, the nurse prescriber should observe if the patients responds to their perceptions. For example, the patients may be looking around the room or actively responding back as if they were having a conversation with another person.

Cognition and memory

People with organic and functional illnesses show signs of cognitive deficit that can be identified at mental state interviews. People with dementia show limitations in short-term and long-term memory. Functional illnesses such as schizophrenia also show progressive cognitive decline in working memory, verbal fluency and attention caused by frequent relapse and prolonged illnesses.

The level of cognition can be assessed by asking patients if they know where they are – time, place and person. Cognition can be further extrapolated by carrying out a mini-mental state examination, which is a 21-item test that gives a good indication of the patient's memory and cognitive state (Folstein *et al.* 1975).

A simple test to examine frontal lobe functioning is to ask the patient to fill in the numbers of a numerical clock face [that you have drawn for them] in the right sequence. Obviously, you would check for any hearing, speech or language deficits before hand.

Verbal fluency can be checked by asking the patient to name 20 words that begin with the letter 'a'. People with cognitive deficits usually score less than 12 within 60 s.

A quick test for abstract thinking may be to ask the patient to explain a simple saying such as 'a rolling stone gathers no moss'. A patient who has difficulties in abstract thinking would explain in concrete terms how stones cannot have moss on them, for example, if they roll down a hill.

When assessing cognitive performance, try to consider the scholastic achievement of the patient and to keep in mind when this achievement was made. For example, it would be clinically relevant to record that a bright high-achieving student suddenly dropped out of university and started to work in a low-paid clerical position.

Attention and concentration

Attention and concentration are different but important aspects. Attention is the ability to apply one's mind to a task, whilst concentration is the ability to sustain one's ability to complete the task. Attention and concentration indices, along with cognition, are particularly relevant for the assessment of older people with functional and organic conditions. Patients who are agitated and depressed may be unable to concentrate on a particular task and so have deficits in remembering what has happened on that day. They may be unable to watch TV because they are *agitated* and recall important news items because they are unable to *concentrate*.

Insight

Mental state examination would not be complete without asking the patients whether they think they are ill or what explanation they give to account for other people's views on their symptoms. At some stage in the patients' journey, they may deny that they are ill or need psychiatric treatment. It is poor practice to just note that a patient has 'no insight' or 'insight lacking'. This is a meaningless statement and should be avoided. Insight also includes asking patients if they would be compliant with treatment. Nurse prescribers may consider particular treatment modalities for patients who display difficulties in accepting they are ill or have poor understanding of the social and vocational aspects of being unwell.

What other assessments can be used?

Mental health nurses have been infused with psycho-social interventions, and they have helped tremendously to bring in a culture of evidence-based assessment tools that help nurses to collect and track psychiatric symptoms (Table 5.1).

The types of assessment chosen depend on what the clinician wishes to find out. The mental state examination identifies what symptoms are present and nurses may delve deeper into the psychopathology to find out the intensity of the symptoms. This is where structured symptom scales are important. Structured scales can also provide a degree of consistency and completeness for the particular illness. Global rating scales are also helpful for the clinician to give a broad assessment of the functioning and result in a single dimension being used to highlight progress.

History and mental state are important, but nurse prescribers must not forget the social aspects and aspirations of patients. Information on how people function and where they live is just as important as the detection and recording of a detailed psychopathology.

Notwithstanding the benefits of the mental state examination, the clinician should be prepared to track the target symptoms that arise from the interview. This may mean that the mental state examination is shortened as the nurse tracks only those symptoms relevant to the examination. The nurse may also supplement the shortened examination by using scales to provide a numerical value (as is their tendency) to the targeted symptoms. The scale can show progress for particular symptoms and whether the treatment is effective. The problem with using a range of symptom scales is the time involved. A mental state examination has an advantage over the various scales in that it is reasonably quick to carry out. It also includes a variety of factors necessary to arrive at a diagnosis and formulation.

Section 3: The consultation

Patients are often worried when they see health professionals. This anxiety is likely to be fuelled when they see nurse prescribers because their expectations will be different when talking to nurses who do not prescribe. The aim of the consultation is to find out what is wrong with them and what is required to help them. The patients must be put at ease as far as practicable, given the

Table 5.1 Assessment scales

Area	Scale	Description	Training required	Comments
Depression	Pierce Suicide Intent Scale	12-item clinician-rated scale	No	Useful for eliciting risk of further attempted suicide
	Becks Depression Inventory (Beck *et al.* 1987)	21-item self-report scale	No	Helpful in detecting the severity of depression
Psychosis	Auditory Hallucinations Rating Scale	11-item clinician-rated scale assessing the frequency, intensity and control over hallucinations	Yes	Useful for tracking of symptoms following a repeated mental state examination
	KGV symptom scale	14-item clinician-rated scale measuring symptoms of schizophrenia	Yes	In-depth assessment process; gives a numerical value
	Delusions Rating Scale (Haddock 1994)	6-item clinician-rated scale assessing presence and intensity of delusions	Yes	Quick tool to track delusional intensity
Mania	Young Mania Rating Scale (Young *et al.* 1978)	11-item clinician-rated scale	Yes	Self-reported symptoms and clinician observations rated over the last 48 h
Global functioning	Global Assessment of Function (Frances *et al.* 1994)	10-item measure of functioning	No	Quick and simple test where the clinician rates the patient against 10 graduated statements
	Camberwell Assessment of Need	22-item clinician-rated scale	Yes	Longer process to identify social deficit
Cognition	Mini-mental state examination (Folstein *et al.* 1975)	21-item clinician-rated scale to measure broad cognitive deficit	No	Quick and simple 'bedside' test
Insight	Insight and Treatment Attitudes Questionnaire (McEvoy *et al.* 1989)	11-item clinician-rated scale to measure three areas of insight	Yes	Scale for assessing insight for schizophrenia. Relies on the interview with patients

circumstance. In order for the nurse prescriber to carry this out, it will be necessary to establish a rapport with the patients. The patients need to be reassured that you are there to take an assessment or review an assessment and that your approach will be based on a nonjudgemental attitude.

The nurse will require particularly developed interpersonal skills like empathy, good eye contact and use of open-ended questions to fully elicit information in order to make the right formulation. This may be difficult or impossible if the patient is aggressive or cognitively confused. For all patients, to establish rapport is the first priority. One way to do this is to initiate the assessment with broad open questions. For example, you could ask 'what has brought you here to see me today' (for a new presentation). Alternatively, you could ask 'we last met a few weeks ago, tell me about any worries you have'. The aim is to enable the patients to trust you and tell you their account.

Good consultations require effective communication. Effective communication is about being able to listen and hearing what is being said during the consultation. It is about showing that you are validating the patient experience. In order for nurse prescribers to be able to listen, they need to be aware of how they greet patients, their body language, where they are sitting and appropriate eye contact. Effective communication is also about being aware of patients' attitudes and being careful to avoid passing judgements on what they are saying or how they are looking or how they are behaving. It is also important to allow patients to speak about what they are experiencing as part of their illness. In order for nurses to do this, nurses need to avoid using closed questions, questions that lead to a 'yes' or a 'no'. Closed questions are useful when clarifying the detail on symptoms or aspects of the history and necessary for clarifying risk assessment.

Open questions – tell me about your symptoms; in what ways they have affected your life? What will help you to take your medication? – are much more fortuitous. It is also important for nurses to check for their understanding of what they are being told and then to drill down, using specific questions, to help the nurse prescriber to decide on what treatment should be prescribed or what interventions used to support the patients to take their medication.

Process of establishing a diagnosis

To perform a diagnosis, nurse prescribers require skills in how to take a history and record a mental state. Although such skills are not beyond nursing, they have not been formally developed within nurse education and are not routinely expected or observed in nursing practice. The debate about the validity and reliability of psychiatric diagnosis will not be had here, albeit to say that diagnosis of conditions is essential for nurse prescribers.

A diagnosis is not just merely giving a name to a list of symptoms. It is about identifying the symptoms that are important and give clues to how the condition developed, its natural course, which treatments work best and the prognosis.

Information gleaned from the history together with the mental state enables the nurse to make a diagnosis. Very often, a provisional diagnosis is made because some clinical situations do not result in cast-iron diagnostic certainty. Nurse prescribers may tend to write a story about the symptoms that can be lengthy and overdescriptive. This is not a bad outcome when nurses first start to chart mental state as long as they differentiate what is recognised pathology by consulting the International Classification of Diseases version 10 (ICD-10) (Cooper 1994). The diagnosis is important for determining what medication, if any, should be offered to patients to alleviate suffering. However, there are a number of caveats about diagnosis that are worth considering here.

When patients present with symptoms, it is important to remember that the symptoms can fall into a number of different categories or clusters. A common example is the symptom of low mood. Low mood occurs in depression, abnormal grief reaction and adjustment disorders. Antidepressant medication may be efficacious for a diagnosed depressive disorder but may not be for an adjustment disorder. This is why nurses should take into account symptoms from the history and the mental state and be able to arrive at the correct diagnosis. Arriving at an incorrect diagnosis carries with it the risk of prescribing a wrong treatment or not prescribing any treatment.

The psychiatric interview may reveal a number of different clusters. For example, the patient may have symptoms of low mood, personality difficulties and alcohol dependence. To help distil the list of symptoms, a range of criteria have been assembled in the ICD-10 so that the nurse can identify the condition from a list of recognised psychiatric disorders. It is worth mentioning that the range of disorders listed in the ICD-10 has been subject to rigorous testing for the reliability and usefulness in clinical practice. If the diagnosis serves no purpose in practice, it is worthless. The nurse takes the list of symptoms collected from the history and from the mental state and goes to the ICD-10 for the broad category heading. The ICD-10 differentiates the disorder into subgroups. By a process of elimination, the clinician sifts through each subtype that best describes the disorder. There are some subtypes that describe the patient as being unspecified.

There is no blood test to prove that the symptoms described by the patient are actually true. Therefore, the interviewer must be able to correctly interpret what the patient is saying and to come up with a clear description of the symptoms.

Patients like to be told their diagnosis and what is wrong with them (Blenkiron 1998). A diagnosis serves as a trading post for patients and nurses to enter into a dialogue about what is wrong with them, what treatments can be offered and what they need to do to keep themselves well. Patient anxieties will require active management. The elicit-provide-elicit strategy is helpful to check for understanding and provide information (Rollnick *et al.* 2000). For example, patients could be informed in simple terms what their diagnosis is and then given pointers to find out more information. The nurse could elicit what information they already have about the condition and then offer them choices to find out more information. Patients are increasingly used to browsing on the Web, accessing self-help manuals and discussing their symptoms with support groups. Some time later, the nurse prescriber then needs to close the loop to check for patient understanding, again eliciting for gaps in knowledge and so on.

To arrive at a working diagnosis is a helpful step in deciding treatment options. However, nurse prescribers need to be mindful that symptoms may become more or less relevant as further history and mental state examination unfolds. A change in diagnosis may then be required. This should be communicated to the patients when this occurs so that they are fully involved with their treatment.

Case summary and formulation

The process of developing a case summary and formulation is a newly developed skill for nurse prescribers. The case summary is extremely important to convey relevant information to the wider team on what has happened to the patient or to convey a review of the case. Nurses may not have to carry out a review every time they see the patient. However, the process of assessment, diagnosis and treatment decisions need to be presented in a way that is accessible and easily understood.

For the formulation, nurses need to start off with writing a brief summary of the problem. The next step is to list a number of possible diagnoses that may be applicable to the presentation. It is important for the nurse to identify the strengths and weaknesses for each diagnosis listed. The nurse then considers what may have caused the disorder in the first place. For example, a patient may present with a depressive disorder and the history confirms that the patient's father suffered from depression and the patient's maternal uncle also took his own life. This genetic predisposition to depression would support the formulation.

It is important for the formulation to include a treatment plan. Treatment may include pharmacological interventions alongside social and psychological interventions carried out by the wider team. For example, a patient was admitted to hospital with a relapse of schizophrenia and responded well to a trial of aripiprazole [drug licensed for the treatment of schizophrenia (BNF 2008)]. The patient experienced less auditory hallucinations and beliefs about people following him in cars subsided. It is clear the patient will require ongoing support at home to identify early warning signs should his condition relapse. Treatment would include specifying the drug, dose and side effects. The patient may be in receipt of social intervention such as support to attend college.

The final step of a formulation is to discuss a prognosis. A badly written formulation gives the clinician little to compare against if the patient goes on to suffer a relapse. For a patient with schizophrenia, who has showed a favourable response to antipsychotic medication, the prognosis would be good if the patient continued to take medication. Social stress would be minimised if the patient engaged well with the community team. Social functioning would be preserved if the patient engaged in vocational activity or paid employment.

Other ways to arrive at a formulation is to consider predisposing, precipitating, perpetuating and protective factors along one axis. Biological factors, psychological elements and social factors would be along the other axis. You then complete the grid for each section (Gelder *et al.* 2004). For example, a predisposing biological factor may be that both parents were diagnosed with early-onset dementia and the patient then presents with what appears to be early-onset cognitive deficits in memory and orientation. A protective social factor may be that the patient lives in a rural setting but very close to family members. One of the sons also resides at home and is willing to look after the patient. Then the formulation is a consideration of all these factors.

Communicating the action plan to patients

How often do patients leave the consultation, not really understanding the medication they have been prescribed? Particularly for patients who are in hospital, satisfaction with information is found to be lacking (Greenwood *et al.* 1999). Nurse prescribers need to make sure that they do not simply replicate any poor-quality prescribing carried out by psychiatrists or the general practitioner. Ways for nurses to improve the quality of prescribing advice is to provide time to the prescribing encounter. When time is lacking, how can nurses provide sufficient information about medicinal products or emotional support to patients who may be anxious about their illness? Nurses are skilled at developing interpersonal relations with patients. However, they may not be so confident in explaining a treatment plan devised by them following an assessment.

The process of taking a history and mental state forges a relationship with the patient. Taking time to collect information on the patient's life story may encourage a willingness to discuss issues that may not have been addressed in the past. The thorough process of a history and mental state examination allows the nurse prescriber to consider a host of factors.

A diagnosis should not be rashly communicated to the patient. Some patients may not be aware of the meaning or go on old-fashioned stereotypes that are completely untrue. It is best to couch a diagnosis on what factors are present and what supports the diagnosis. The intention is not to be ambiguous. One way for nurses to approach this is to discuss with the patient their signs and symptoms. This not only checks the accuracy of the assessment process but also displays to patients that you understand their symptoms. The formulation process described above serves as a useful framework to discuss a diagnosis.

User groups produce information booklets about the diagnosis that present the information in plain English so that the right impression is put across. You will need to convey to the patient the course and prognosis of their condition and likely treatment options. People with mental health problems, particularly those individuals affected by habitual substance misuse, may find the traditional format of written information difficult to take on board. Examples of patients being given information via a podcast and video diaries have been piloted with some success (National Prescribing Centre 2008).

It will take time for the patient to understand the implications of their diagnosis. Nurses will need to check for understanding and should be willing to invest time in explaining the diagnosis and what it means for them.

Explaining the treatment plan goes beyond simply telling the patient they are on a type of medication, with a list of reasons why they should take it. Chapter 8 discusses this in depth and clearly illustrates how nurses can work with patients to achieve partnership in medicines management.

Providing care to people is more than just diagnosing the condition and prescribing medication. It is also about explaining to the patient the range of services that are available to them. Part of this care may be for the patient to consider any legal advice or advocacy.

When medication is discussed with the patient, it is helpful to provide written information on the drug itself, along with information about its side effects. It is important that nurse prescribers provide patients with the full range of information that is available on medicines. This helps the patient to buy into the taking of their prescribed medication and make informed choices.

A question that is often asked by patients at the end of an inpatient stay or a consultation is whether they can drive or work. The answer depends on the medication prescribed and how well the patient is. For driving, responsibility is on the patient to inform their insurance company if medical circumstances change and this includes the prescribing of psychotropic medication. Prescribers have a responsibility to inform the patient that certain medication has the potential to affect driving (Taylor *et al.* 2007). Generally, patients need to be 'well' for at least 3 months after they leave hospital, before they can drive.

Conclusion

Both the history and mental state examination should not be seen as isolated and detached processes. It is important that the history and mental state examination is recorded accurately at the time of taking the information. It is surprising how much information is lost if notes are not taken contemporaneously. Nurses will not be familiar with the practice of contemporaneous note taking, which is a skill to be learnt. The assessment process covered in this chapter has attempted to cover relevant issues for adults, older people and substance misuse services. This quite clearly shows that the process of taking a history needs to be purposeful and adapted for each individual patient for assessment. Each specialty will have in-depth questions that drop down from these core areas. Other assessment tools to detect the extent of conviction in abnormal beliefs and the extent of cognitive impairment should also be used if deemed clinically relevant. Certainly, the process of symptom tracking can be enhanced by particular tools, but they take time to complete and offer the formulation greater depth and meaning.

Chapter 6
Coexisting medical conditions

Introduction

The mortality and morbidity rates for people with mental health problems are a public health scandal. Current estimates suggest that people with schizophrenia die 10 years earlier than the general population (Brown 1997). People who have schizophrenia, bipolar disorder and depression have a higher incidence of heart disease, stroke and diabetes compared to people without these conditions (Disability Rights Commission 2006, Farmer *et al.* 2008). People who have mental health problems may be discriminated against receiving assessment and treatment for their medical conditions because of their mental health problem diagnosis (DoH 2006d). They may well receive the most up-to-date treatment for their mental health problems but the outcomes of conditions that shorten the life of patients such as coronary heart disease (CHD) and diabetes receive scant attention (Connolly & Kelly 2005).

In this chapter, the major medical conditions that commonly coexist within the broad family of mental health will be discussed. A nurse prescriber will need to take on board coexisting medical conditions because the prescribing of medication may be altered by how the condition affects metabolism or excretion of the drug from the body. Nurse prescribers will also be in an ideal position to screen and then refer to specialist teams for advice and intervention for a patient. Much of this work should be performed in primary care. Many nurses work in primary care and are in an ideal position to carry out these investigations and act on them themselves.

Nurse prescribers can make a significant impact on improving overall health by being mindful of coexisting medical conditions. Targeted symptom tracking may reduce healthcare costs further down the chain. It is important to remember that maintaining stability in a patient's mental health is the first step to helping the patient take control over their physical health.

Health promotion is a key role for nurse prescribers and should be practised in the settings where nurses work and deliver their interventions. Hence, opportunities should be exploited so that health promotion can be delivered as part of an integrated approach. All areas of mental health would be ideal for all-round health promotion strategies.

Dual diagnosis

Alcohol use across the world has been identified as a major cause of mortality and morbidity and thus accounts for 3% of all deaths (World Health

Organisation 2002). It is recognised that people with serious mental health problems use drugs and alcohol to harmful levels causing harm to themselves, families and others. The problem appears to worsen if the patient lives in an urban area (36%) (Menezes *et al.* 1996). Alcohol misuse also increases criminal justice costs as well as reduced work productivity in society (Anderson & Baumberg 2006). Poly-drug misuse within the population is also rising. An Irish study found that the possible reason for increased alcohol consumption with heroin may be the substitution of one drug for another in the belief that it has less damage (MacManus & Fitzpatrick 2007).

For these reasons alone, nurse prescribers need to be proficient in the taking of an alcohol and drug history. The aim is to consider what impact this has on the prescribed medication. For example, people who take heroin may be more at risk by the prescription of methadone.

Metabolic syndrome

There are a group of disorders that fall under the umbrella of metabolic syndrome. This is central obesity and this factor is accompanied by two of the following four conditions: raised triglyceride levels, reduced high-density lipoprotein, raised blood pressure, raised fasting blood glucose (Zimmet *et al.* 2005). These conditions seriously worsen health outcomes for conditions such as schizophrenia (Brown *et al.* 2000). Evidence points towards the emergence of metabolic syndrome with the presence of medication to treat psychotic disorders such as schizophrenia and mood disorder (Ryan & Thakore 2002). Most antipsychotic medication is linked to the rise in obesity for people with schizophrenia, but drugs that come under the class of dibenzodiazepines, such as clozapine and olanzapine, are particularly worse (Stahl 2006).

Coronary heart disease

People with mental health problems are more likely to have CHD. Rates for hypertension are 34% vs 29% for the general population. Hypertension increases the risk of cardiovascular disease. Average systolic pressure is more than 135 mmHg and a diastolic greater than 85 mmHg (Joint British Society 2005). Psychiatric drug treatment may worsen these indices resulting in hypertension. Nurse prescribers need to be aware of referring on patients when systolic pressure rises above these indices because medication may be required. However, nurse prescribers can persuade the patient to engage in lifestyle modification including weight management and 30 min of exercise daily.

Psychiatric medication alters the electrical rhythm of the cardiac cycle. This is why nurse prescribers should take an electrocardiogram when patients are admitted into hospital or when certain medication is likely to be prescribed or medication is to be prescribed to a high level. The 12 lead electrocardiogram report will provide important information that all nurses will find essential such as the rate of the cardiac cycle and the QTc interval. In men, the QTc should not exceed 450 ms, and in women, 470 ms. Serious note should be given to readings when the QTc exceeds 500 ms and a decision should be made to refer the patient to a cardiologist for an opinion on starting or continuing with the current medication (Welch & Chue 2000).

Diabetes

In the UK, up to 5% of people have type 2 diabetes, which is a condition where there is decreased sensitivity to insulin. Type 1 diabetes is where the pancreas does not secrete any insulin. Up to 20% of people with schizophrenia suffer from type 2 diabetes (Gough & O'Donovan 2005). Psychotropic medication is linked with impaired glucose metabolism (Bushe & Leonard 2004). Surprisingly, a large study in the USA of 38 632 patients found that people taking atypical drugs such as clozapine and olanzapine were 9% more likely to have diabetes than those patients taking the older typical neuroleptic drugs (Sernyak *et al.* 2002).

Obesity is a risk factor for diabetes, and psychotropic-induced weight gain is a major factor (Sussman 2001). Other factors such as a family predisposition, increasing longevity and ethnicity are important (Connolly & Kelly 2005). Diabetes results in a number of macrocomplications and microcomplications such as visual impairment or amputation as a result of impaired circulation. Unexplained weight loss, polyuria and polidypsia are the classic tell-tale signs for diabetes. Diabetes can be delayed and prevented by the change in lifestyle, such as diet and exercise. This is where self-management becomes important. Patients need to be offered information that leads them to make the choices to take control over their lifestyle. However, for people who have mental health problems, this control may not be so easy.

Interventions to be carried out by a nurse prescriber should include routine monitoring of plasma glucose levels. Monitoring of HbA1c indicates whether glycemic control is being managed. This is an important marker because it indicates the mean blood glucose level over the last 3 months ($\leqslant$7%). When this marker rises above 8%, active treatment, medication or change in medication is required. Nurse prescribers need to be aware that diabetes is a chronic condition that not only requires self-management by a patient but also service-level monitoring.

Obesity and malnutrition

Life expectancy is reduced by 9 years simply by being obese. Obesity results in 30 000 deaths per annum in the UK (Holt 2005) and accounts for 1.5% of NHS expenditure (National Audit Office 2001). Obesity is a growing problem in the UK, but it is particularly serious for people with mental health problems. At a body mass index greater than $25\,kg/m^2$, it increases the risk of developing other metabolic disorders such as diabetes, CHD and dyslipidaemia (Ryan & Thakore 2002).

Weight indices are an imprecise method to estimate problems. The body mass index is a calculation of whether a person is in a healthy weight range for their height. The body mass index is also a predictor in terms of the risk of developing coexisting medical conditions (World Health Organisation 2007). For example, patients who have a body mass index greater than $27\,kg/m^2$ may be at an increased risk to develop heart disease, diabetes or hypertension, or have impaired lipids. Nurse prescribers can also use a tape measure to record hip and waist circumference by asking the patient to stand in a relaxed posture after breathing out (National Obesity Forum 2008).

Obesity is higher in females with schizophrenia, rising to 71% (Dickerson *et al.* 2002). This is the reason why nurse prescribers need to carry out regular weight checks, discuss diet, do exercise, and take lipid profiles. People with schizophrenia are less likely to exercise and opt for unhealthy food choices (McCreadie 2003).

Nurse prescribers need to be aware that medication may be related to weight gain. Almost all of the antipsychotic medication leads to weight gain, some much more than the others. An example is olanzapine versus aripiprazole, the former having a higher propensity for weight gain (Taylor *et al.* 2007). Agents such as aripiprazole have less effect on weight gain, hence aripiprazole has potential therapeutic effect in the treatment of schizophrenia and bipolar disorder (Chrzanowski *et al.* 2006).

Weight gain associated with depot antipsychotic medication has been found to be a major factor towards discontinuation of medication and relapse (Silverstone *et al.* 1988).

Dyslipidaemia

Cholesterol in the blood is a predictor of CHD (Young 2005). It is important to monitor lipid levels because people treated with antipsychotic medication showed a threefold increase in cholesterol (Saari *et al.* 2004). Evidence suggests that a lowering of cholesterol reduces the risk of CHD. The total amount of cholesterol is made up of a number of fractions; the most important of these is low-density lipoprotein. Low-density lipoprotein is involved in plaque formation in the coronary arteries leading to a cardiovascular event such as a stroke or a heart attack. High-density lipoprotein acts as a protective element (Assmann *et al.* 1996). Triglyceride levels are also an independent risk factor for CHD. The tragedy however is that people with mental health problems are often overlooked in the treatment of this modifiable risk factor (Hennekens *et al.* 2005).

Respiratory conditions

Smoking is habit forming and occurs much more frequently in people with mental health problems. Smoking increases the risk of developing chronic obstructive pulmonary disease. The tell-tale signs for chronic obstructive airways disease include a chronic cough, production of sputum and breathlessness upon exercise. People who have serious mental health problems have an increased risk of developing respiratory conditions such as chronic bronchitis (19% vs 6%) and emphysema (8% vs 1.5%) (Himelhoch *et al.* 2004). Patients may also require treatment with antibiotics to treat the range of respiratory conditions. Nurse prescribers may rely on the diagnosis from junior medical staff or from general practitioners.

Patients susceptible to developing or who have influenza need to be prompted to visit their general practitioner for annual influenza immunisation. Patients should be prompted to seek quick attention when they develop respiratory infections. A range of psychotropic medication can reduce respiratory rate. For example diazepam [drug licensed for anxiety (BNF 2008)] can suppress respiratory rate.

Asthma is a common respiratory condition; many patients do not attend to this condition and the result is a worsening of the condition. The goal for managing asthma is to reduce the frequency of symptoms, which range from wheezing, tightness in the chest to shortness of breath. Nurse prescribers need to monitor the frequency of symptoms and how often patients use their inhaler.

Pregnancy

Pregnancy is not a medical condition but it is a vital consideration for the prescribing of drugs if women are of child-bearing age, thinking of starting a family, have unprotected sex or who are pregnant (Usher *et al.* 2005). There is a lack of long-term evidence examining new drugs, which is why older drugs like haloperidol are considered for people with psychotic conditions. Some drugs such as valproate [drug licensed for bipolar disorder (BNF 2008)] are known to be harmful to the developing foetus and should be avoided (NICE 2006c). Prescribing for women who are pregnant requires extensive medical knowledge and experience and would fall outside the current skill set of nurse prescribers. Advice would be to transfer care back to the psychiatrist or general practitioner in these circumstances.

Smoking

Smoking is a social and pharmacological addiction but certain populations engage in smoking more than the others. These not only include people with mental health problems but also those who are in lower social classes. Seventy per cent of people with schizophrenia are addicted to nicotine (McCreadie 2003) and this is striking when compared to 20% of the smoking population. Smoking is one of the most documented health hazards and interventions should be adopted that tackle this addiction (Connolly & Kelly 2005). Nicotine addiction is responsible for a host of diseases and conditions such as cardiovascular disease, a range of cancers and respiratory conditions (NICE 2008).

Smoking has implications for the prescription of medication. More medication may be needed as the action of smoking increases the rate of liver metabolism. Nurse prescribers need to be aware of the medications that increase metabolism and what impact smoking cessation would have on mental state (see Table 6.1).

Smoking cessation programmes have been found to have good effect in mental health and substance misuse populations (Rice & Stead 2008). The link between stopping smoking and the risk of relapse towards alcohol misuse is unfounded (Cooney *et al.* 2003). People who stop smoking but continue to take methadone also tend to use less illicit substances (Shoptaw *et al.* 2002). The game plan should be for nurses to offer opportunities for patients to discuss their smoking habit, and intentions to give up. Evidence supporting smoking

Table 6.1 Effects of psychotropic medication for smokers

Drug	Action of smoking	Effect of smoking cessation on serum concentrations	What to do with current medication if giving nicotine replacement therapy
Diazepam	Smoking stimulates CNS, hence reduce hypnotic effect	Patients may report increased sedation	Reduce the dose
Chlorpromazine	Reduces serum concentrations	Patients may report increased EPSE	Reduce the dose
Clozapine	Reduces serum concentrations by 50%	Patients report increased sedation and hypotensive effect	Reduce the dose
Haloperidol	Reduces serum concentrations by 20%	Patients report increased EPSE	Reduce the dose
Olanzapine	Reduces serum concentrations by 50% and can reduce efficacy on symptoms	Increased risk of metabolic syndrome	Reduce the dose
Lithium	Slows excretion rate of lithium	Increases xanthine levels, therefore increases lithium excretion	Monitor lithium levels more frequently

Sources: North West Medicines Information Centre (2006); Jones & Jones (2008a); Taylor *et al.* (2007); Bazire (2007); and Carrillo *et al.* (2003).
CNS, central nervous system; EPSE, extrapyramidal side effect.

cessation activities is growing; particularly when motivational groups coupled with nicotine replacement are delivered in combination (Ranney *et al.* 2006).

The advice for nurses is to target those people who have mental health problems and belong to hard-to-reach communities, ethnic minority groups and socio-economically disadvantaged groups of society (NICE 2008). Targets are put forward such as success rates of 35% at a week 4 quit date. Interventions to work alongside pharmacology include behavioural counselling on a one-to-one basis, group delivery or interventions delivered as part of the intervention.

Infections

People who engage in high-risk behaviours such as injecting drugs are susceptible to health problems such as hepatitis C virus (HCV) and human immunodeficiency virus (HIV) infections. This health epidemic will have long-lasting morbidity and mortal implications for the foreseeable future without early and consistent intervention and education.

HCV is one of the most common blood borne infections. Up to 15% of hepatitis C will develop a cirrhotic liver and up to 4% will develop liver cancer. People who inject drugs carry the highest risk of contracting hepatitis C. Patients can also be referred to the general practitioner for immunisation against hepatitis A and B.

People who inject heroin may require information about rival HCV and HIV infections. Patients may have concerns about the likely treatment and prognosis for hepatitis C. For example, patients can be informed about behaviour and lifestyle changes. Alcohol consumption, for example, increases the rate of HIV infection (Freeman *et al.* 2001). Smoking tobacco reduces the efficacy of treatment for interferon (El-Zayadi 2006).

Hepatic and renal disorders

People with mental health problems misuse alcohol and drugs to excess leading to impaired liver function. Ten per cent of people who have been prescribed antipsychotic medication have impaired liver function (Garcia-Unzueta *et al.* 2003). The liver metabolises drugs, and if it is impaired, then the rate of metabolism may be reduced because the drug accumulates more readily. Under these conditions the amount of drug to be prescribed would have to be reduced, thus affecting efficacy. Nurses need to be mindful that a patient presenting with a normal range of liver function tests may still have hepatic disease.

One study has estimated that 6.5% of people referred for service present with an abnormal renal function (Duncan *et al.* 2001). Renal impairment can be directly measured by how well the kidneys filter the blood by using a ratio called the glomerular filtration rate (GFR). A normal GFR is $90\,ml/min/1.73\,m^2$. A GFR of $59\,ml/min/1.73\,m^2$ indicates moderate impairment and so the nurse would check what impact certain drugs have on the kidneys (Taylor *et al.* 2007).

At the very least, nurses need to understand the principles of how the kidneys excrete drugs and the various stages of renal impairment. Prescribing for older people would automatically register a potentially impaired GFR. The kidneys may not be able to filter the blood to remove the drug adequately, leading to an increased accumulation of the drug itself or its metabolites. Nurse prescribers need to have knowledge of certain drugs that are toxic to the kidneys, such as lithium, and that lithium is to be avoided in circumstances where the patient has more than mild renal impairment.

Sexual health

Patients may be concerned about their ability to form relationships or to practice sex safely. Substance abusers may have worries about having children or coping with the burdens of being a parent. HIV and HCV may also be transmitted to the unborn child; therefore, nurses will need to offer advice about sexual health to prevent pregnancy. Alternatively, the nurse may need to refer to specialist advice if pregnancy is sought.

Sexual health may be affected by endocrine factors associated with psychotropic medication. Certain dopaminergic drugs raise the level of prolactin, thus mimicking the effects of pregnancy. A potent atypical antipsychotic drug that causes raised prolactin is amisulpride (BNF 2008). Prolactin is a hormone and its primary function is to bring on lactation in females (Wieck & Haddad 2003). Elevation can affect menstrual cycle producing oligorrhoea and amenorrhoea. On a long-term basis, the condition causes abnormal bone density deposits in women (Meaney & O'Keane 2002). Other drugs affect alpha-1 receptors and so affect libido and the ability to sustain a sexual arousal and ejaculatory response. Nurse prescribers need to be able to carry out a sexual history and to consider the effects that medication may have on sexual functioning.

Interventions to manage coexisting medical conditions

It is important for nurse prescribers to have skills in facilitating groups and deliver practicable investigations that can tackle health inequalities such as diabetes and heart disease. It is important to keep in mind that the excess rates of chronic diseases can be reduced with concerted effort. Well-being programmes have been developed that give patients information about the condition and strategies to help them having control over their lifestyle. Nurses need to adopt health promotion strategies that target the wider determinants of health, covering awareness and access to primary care services, strategies to reduce alcohol and substance misuse and nicotine cessation (Brimblecombe *et al.* 2007).

When patients present to service or they have their medication reviewed, nurse prescribers need to consider the risks of developing coexisting medical conditions. An evaluation of living, lifestyle and the risk of medication contributing towards or worsening medical conditions need to be considered. A change in medication in the face of a coexisting medical condition should not always be the first consideration.

Better nutrition

When we think of nutrition, the first aspect that comes to mind is overeating or undereating. These are important clinical features of mental health problems or a coexisting medical condition. The link between nutrition and mental health is also important in terms of what people eat and how they can eat a diet richer in certain types of fats such as fish for the omega-3 content (Food Health Forum 2008).

Evidence is emerging of a link between poor nutritional content and increasing rates of depression, particularly self-harm (Garland *et al.* 2007) and suicide (Tanskanen *et al.* 2001). People who have a first episode of psychosis receive less antipsychotic medication when they are given omega-3 capsules (Berger *et al.* 2004). There is a level of evidence that omega-3 adds a protective element against developing dementia but the results are not conclusive (Lim *et al.* 2006). It is now recommended that mental health services set up clinics to assess nutritional content and draw up care plans to meet this need for people with mental health problems. Nurse prescribers should be part of or establish links with these clinics given the potential to prescribe omega-3 for psychiatric patients.

Nurses can help patients to control obesity, and the first step is for the patient to loose weight (Wirshing *et al.* 2003). Control over weight in people with schizophrenia has been associated with improved health outcomes. A 5% reduction in weight can positively improve morbidity and mortality indices including glucose control (Institute of Medicine 1995). Nurse prescribers should consider setting up wellness clinics to take stock of a patient's level of exercise per week, diet and habits for eating. Patients can then be advised to lower the amount of calories they eat and to take up a regular exercise pattern. Evidence shows that reducing the amount of calories that a patient takes coupled with physical exercise will reduce weight (Wu *et al.* 2007).

Some people may not have learnt how to adopt a regular exercise pattern or may find it difficult to establish links with their neighbourhood. Nurses can consider running exercise classes that go through the steps of accessing the local gym and local walking groups and organising walking trips to local areas. Support may come from practicable interventions such as picking up patients and taking them to the gym. Support may be gained from their peers.

In some organisations, it is not just nurses who are interested in the health benefits of weight reduction. Dieticians can be asked to form a collaborative agreement with mental health organisations so that the added skills from these professions can be used to good effect (O'Keefe *et al.* 2003). Dieticians, for example, can be asked to construct cal-orie diets that reduce intake over a 3-month period. Assessments can be made of the types of foodstuffs that patients eat and to find ways for healthy options to be built into the weekly eating habits. For example, we know that people with schizophrenia have the tendency to have a poor diet and do less exercise (McCreadie *et al.* 1998).

Improvement in diets can be made using more fresh fruit and vegetables in meals, sugar-free foods and drinks and less processed ready-made meals. Some studies have shown that providing patients with fruit and vegetables does result in more intake. As soon as this intervention is stopped, patients return to base-line levels of intake (McCreadie *et al.* 2005). What this shows is that simply providing advice or food is not enough. Patients need to make the link and be motivated to change their dietary habits, which may have been embedded for many years.

Occupational therapists can help patients to structure a functional day that includes a minimum of 30 minutes of daily activity. Helping patients to struc-ture their day is necessary because patients with schizophrenia often display symptoms of disorganisation. Motivation to reduce weight may also be difficult as again this is impaired for people with depression and psychotic conditions. Important points to consider are ensuring the exercise actually does no harm to the patient or does not incur expense to already small budgets. Walking seems the ideal exercise programme. Daumit *et al.* (2005) found that for people with serious mental health problems, walking is the most common form of exercise.

Exercise can obviously take many forms, such as brisk walking, walking up and down the stairs in the house and more formalised exercise regimens such as circuit training in the local gym. The recommended amount of exercise is 30 min of brisk exercise every day. The aim of exercise is to cancel out the amount of calories taken by the body and thereby burn off fat. Safe reduction of weight should occur at a rate of 0.5–1.0 kg per week. It is not just the prescription of medication that should take place but also the prescription of exercise.

The overall aim of interventions targeted at obese people is to:

- reduce body mass index;
- lower the harmful body fats;
- lower waist–hip percentage.

Substance misuse

There is a wide-ranging policy mix to address substance misuse across the UK (DoH 2002). People who misuse substance are socially excluded from main-stream activities such as recreation, suitable accommodation and support services for themselves (Kavanagh *et al.* 2000). Evidence supports the role of training clinicians in dual diagnosis to improve service outcomes (Munro *et al.* 2007). Priority areas include a drive on helping people to reduce or resist temp-tation to use drugs and alcohol. This should be carried out in a nonpunitive fashion and be individually tailored. Examples are harm reduction strategies that help to minimise the amount of drug taken and to safeguard young families from the trauma of living with people who take drugs.

Women who drink more than 35 units of alcohol per week and men 50 units of alcohol per week are at a high risk of alcohol-related comorbidity (DoH 2007c). A simple strategy for alcohol misuse that can be used by nurse prescribers would be to increase people's awareness of how much they drink and what are 'safe' limits. The strategy would be to build in days when the patient does not take alcohol and avoid the social or expected norm to 'binge' drink. Nurse prescribers can also use harm reduction strategies. The aim is to help the patient use harm reduction strategies (Lenton & Single 1998). The strength of the approach is that it does not focus on abstinence and tends to be more pragmatic in clinical practice. The central point is to guide the patient to think about the risks of alcohol and how these could be lessened.

Health services have great potential to support patients to reduce alcohol consumption. Patients may enter accident and emergency departments, visit general practitioners or wider primary care services, or may be supported in specialist mental health services. Brief motivational interviewing techniques can be used to reduce alcohol consumption and alcohol-related injuries. Patients can also be supported to abstain through interventions delivered through the Internet (Saitz *et al.* 2007).

Smoking cessation

Nurse prescribers must use every intervention or patient contact as an opportunity to persuade and encourage patients to stop smoking. Guidelines have been developed to give the nurse a framework for this to take place (Rigotti *et al.* 2001). However, nurse prescribers must bear in mind that diagnosis itself is not the only consideration. Factors such as age, gender, class, ethnicity and pregnancy all play a part in the receptivity of smoking advice (NICE 2008). Box 6.1

Box 6.1   Smoking cessation intervention that can be delivered by nurse prescribers.

Step 1
Patients should be asked about their nicotine consumption and this should be recorded. For example, how many cigarettes smoked per day and when they smoke them.

Step 2
Patients should be advised on the advantages of stopping smoking. One way would be to link the advantage directly to the personal circumstances of the patient. For example, people with depression may be unable to work and be short on money. Saving the money spent on cigarettes can be used to pay outstanding debts or bills.

Step 3
Patients should be assessed on the willingness to give up smoking and what are the barriers to its cessation. One way would be to ask the patient to set a cessation date in the next 30 days and what steps they would take to achieve this.
Step 3 also involves an assessment of smoking cessation intervention and what the patient's preference would be.

Step 4

This stage is really important because patients are assisted to give up smoking through the use of medication and motivational interviewing and support groups. Types of pharmacotherapy include nicotine replacement and partial agonists. Support groups can be run from clinics, hospitals and community centres, or even over the telephone.

Step 5

People who receive case management will be seen again. Part of the consultation is to include a review of the smoking cessation intervention.

---

lists the 10-min consultation advice that has been adapted from Koplan *et al.* (2008).

The beauty about this five-step programme is that it can be delivered by any health professional and can be delivered quickly as part of usual care and treatment within mental health services. The only barrier to implementation is the way smoking is perceived within the culture of mental health services.

Patients should be asked if they would like to have smoking cessation advice from a trained counsellor in individual sessions or as part of a group. The end message here is that nurse prescribers should be fully aware of how to deliver short blasts of smoking cessation advice as well as being aware of how to refer to specialist cessation services.

Caffeine

Many foodstuffs such as Coca-Cola and other juice drinks contain added caffeine. The mean caffeine intake per day in the UK is between 350 and 620 mg (Rihs *et al.* 1996). However, it would be fairly uncommon for nurse prescribers to take account of the amount of caffeine patients consume.

Caffeine is absorbed through the gut, metabolised in the liver and excreted through the kidneys. Caffeine antagonises adenosine receptors. When adenosine receptors become blocked with excessive caffeine use, this can lead to palpitations and cardiac dysrhythmia. People can also experience increased anxiety, insomnia and agitation. Caffeine can affect the metabolism of various psychotropic drugs by competing for the metabolic pathways, an example is of clozapine prescribed for schizophrenia (Carillo *et al.* 1998) and benzodiazepines for anxiety disorders (Bruce 1990).

Nurse prescribers should be mindful to ask about caffeine consumption, and if this is in excess, they should distinguish symptoms of excess from other mental health problems. A clinical example is to ask about sleep. One cup of brewed coffee equals 136 mg of caffeine, but only 200 mg is required to affect the sleep and disrupt the sleep cycles (Fredholm *et al.* 1999). The heart of assessment is to take a nutritional history and when caffeine intake rises above 250 mg per day to offer intervention.

Table 6.2 Caffeine sources and content

Source	Caffeine content
Cup of tea (T-bag)	50 mg
Cup of tea (brewed in pot)	40 mg
Cup of green tea	30 mg
Cup of brewed coffee	100–136 mg
Cup of instant coffee	60–95 mg
Plain chocolate bar	50 mg
Coca-Cola (can)	40 mg

Source: Taylor *et al.* (2007); Food Standards Agency (2004).

When patients take caffeine more than 600 mg per day, it can produce psycho-motor problems, insomnia and disorientation (Sawynok 1995). Some patients may be unable to remember the amount of caffeine intake and so one solution may be a drink diary completed over 2 weeks. Nurse prescribers will need to be able to calculate how much of caffeine is present in each drink to arrive at a cumulative total (Table 6.2).

Nurse prescribers need to remember that stopping high intakes of caffeine can produce withdrawal such as headaches and low mood (Silverman *et al.* 1992). Abrupt cessation will also affect the bioavailability of some psychotropic drugs and therefore lead to more side effects or a heightened effect of the drug.

Conclusion

The overall message from this chapter is that people with mental health and substance misuse problems do carry a higher risk of developing or having coexisting medical problems. Routine assessment of these problems is necessary if nurses are to embrace the full agenda with nurse prescribing. Nurses need to be aware that the medication they prescribe may actually induce and worsen the range of medical conditions listed above. This calls for training to be able to take and understand the consequences of a medical history plus the ability to detect changes in endocrine and metabolic indices over time.

Nurse prescribers are in an ideal position to take on board the huge public health agenda for people facing mental health problems. The process of taking a medical history (as part of full history-taking process) will indicate areas where people are at risk of developing metabolic syndrome or other coexisting medical conditions. There is a deficit in health promotion activities and many of our interventions occur when the condition has been diagnosed.

This is why it is very important for nurse prescribers to not only raise their own awareness but also that of others regarding the risks of coexisting medical conditions. Screening and ongoing monitoring are therefore essential to complement informed prescribing decisions. It is clear from this chapter that nurses should seek to provide assessment that cover mental health, addiction and physical health. The problem is that people with mental health problems may be less organised to go about seeking intervention. They may be resistive to health intervention through social or cognitive decline. Herein lays the challenge for nurses to take on board the public health agenda and make physical health the core business within nurse prescribing.

Chapter 7
Nurse prescribing in the real world

Introduction

The aim of this chapter is to help clinicians to implement prescriptive authority and to show how nurse prescribing can be used in particular service settings. Nurse prescribing requires an environment where nurses are able to develop their newly developed skills. Indeed nurse prescribing has helped to shape new roles such as advanced nurse practitioners and nurse consultants. We have also seen the advent of nurse-led services where nurses are managing groups of patients with similar types of needs who require standard sets of interventions on a regular basis. Nurses are also working in specialist teams. Almost all areas are suitable for nurse prescribing and what is required is a mindset and organisational will to put it into practice.

How could nurse prescribing work in practice: Service settings

There are many service settings where nurse prescribing can work (see Table 7.1).

Table 7.1 Areas where nurse prescribing could offer advantages to patients and the service redesign agenda

Areas	Advantages
Emergency care	Meet 4-h accident and emergency waiting time
General practice and primary care	Expand capacity to meet increasing demand
Hospital at night schemes	Meet European Working Time Directive changes for junior doctors
Sexual health clinics	The actual relationship with patients may bring about longer term contact
Prison healthcare units	Increase outreach capacity to this underserved community
Nurse-led clinics	Make better use of psychiatrist skills
Hospital wards	Medication partnerships with patients and increase capacity within the team

Primary care and primary care mental health services

The opportunity for community psychiatric nurses and practice nurses to develop prescribing skills in the primary care environment is tremendous.

Ninety per cent of mental health care is provided in a primary care setting and the majority of people experience anxiety and depressive disorders (Goldberg & Huxley 1992). Primary care is often seen as a general practitioner working in a surgery with district nurses and practice nurses. Primary care has now expanded into health centres, walk-in centres and polyclinics.

There are an increasing number of people with severe mental illness who are cared for within primary care, with minimal or no input from secondary services (Goldberg & Huxley 1992). The opportunity for nurse prescribers to work up practice-based serious mental illness registers for the management of medication and physical health monitoring is vast.

Nurse-led clinics

The evidence supporting nurse-led clinics is developing rapidly, particularly around concordance and satisfaction with care (Ridsdale 1997; Wong & Chung 2006) and the health promotion role (Hatchett 2003). Nurse-led clinics first started in the 1980s in areas of physical medicine, such as diabetes. There are many examples of mental health clinics where nurse prescribers work, such as memory clinics (Barlow *et al.* 2008) and clozapine clinics (Leppard 2008). Clinics most often are focused towards people who have chronic conditions that have been diagnosed by a doctor. However, there is scope to broaden out the concept of nurse-led clinics and to focus on acute care or to diagnose conditions not previously seen.

The language to describe nurse-led care assumes that patients are only seen by nursing staff without any medical oversight or reference to the multidisciplinary team. Nothing could be further from the truth for effective team working. Clinics are part of primary and secondary care and function to meet the needs of a particular service.

The development of nurse-led care requires a reordering of who does what across the pathway. This will most often require a challenge to established norms of practice. Nurse-led clinics can support psychiatrists in the delivery of community care and to siphon those patients who do not need to be seen by a psychiatrist. The reduced psychiatrist time could then be used for those patients who require urgent and intense medical input, clinical training and supervision for nurses.

The expansion of nurse-led clinics will raise to the surface the issues relating to the nursing profession. Nurses will need to consider how and where growth in the system will occur. Areas for expansion may be health centres, community centres or arrangements with the voluntary sector. This is echoed by the latest Chief Nursing Officer report (DoH 2006c) that supports the direction of travel for nurses to take on the management of long-term conditions as part of a whole team and service development. Foundation trusts (National Health Service organisations with more autonomy from the central government) will certainly examine the cost realisation of developing nurse-led services.

Secondary care community teams

To differentiate between primary and secondary care can be arbitrary at times, but for the purposes of this discussion, secondary care can include community mental health teams, assertive outreach teams and home treatment teams. Mental health nurses are key members both in the number and in the role they play in the functioning of these teams. The potential for nurses to use prescribing skills is immense. It seems logical for organisations to invest in nurses to acquire prescribing skills.

Community mental health teams remain a core element of an integrated secondary care service for people with serious mental illness. Community psychiatric nurses could prescribe medication more easily for people when they visit them at home, particularly at junctures such as careful titration of medication. For services without a nurse prescriber, usually, a change in medication would require a conversation and agreement with the psychiatrist or the general practitioner. This may not always happen quickly, thus resulting in delay and further distress to the patient.

Assertive outreach teams aim to develop therapeutic relationships with patients who are difficult to engage with community services (DoH 1999c). A core element of assertive outreach is medication concordance. Nurse prescribers working in such teams may have a greater chance of medication concordance with the patient than a psychiatrist who only sees the patient once every 3 months.

A similar argument can be made for home treatment teams. The window of opportunity to initiate and sustain concordance is when people are unwell. Nurses will often be professionals who are at the front end of assessment and home treatment. Building in nurse prescribers into home treatment teams will enable services more to meet service user demand but also offer a more consistent patient-driven agenda in terms of symptom resolution.

Psychiatric hospital care

Hospital processes require continual readjustment because of the costs and the high-risk nature of the environment. Patients also have concerns about the level of engagement with staff, when they are admitted to hospital (Sainsbury Centre for Mental Health 2005). Nurse prescribing may bring about some remedy to this situation, along with other socially inclusive and safety-focused interventions.

A question posed by some may be whether nurse prescribing has any role in hospital settings, given the availability of doctors. This is a wrong conclusion, as nurse prescribing was never about replacing doctors. Research and anecdotal commentaries suggest that hospital services may be appropriate for prescribing activity and may provide an opportunity for career development and advancement in skills (Jones 2006c,d; Murray 2007). Potential exists for some experienced nurses, such as nurse consultants, to provide 'cover' for psych-iatrists when they are on annual leave (Jones & Harborne 2005; Jones & Jones 2006). Models of implementation are emerging that stress the interdependency between the nurse prescriber and the psychiatrist when using supplementary prescribing on hospital wards. The role of the psychiatrist would be to guide the clinical practice of the team, seeing some patients when difficulties arise but, for the most part, acting as the consultant to the team. The nurse prescriber works as part of the team dealing with some patients in full and, for others, under the direction of the psychiatrist (Jones 2006a; Harborne & Jones 2008).

Potential sources of conflict for this model would include difficulties in dif-ferentiating the role of junior medical staff from that of the nurse prescriber and in deciding who would hold responsibility for monitoring patient care within the confines of a clinical management plan. Of more importance, and borne out in the literature, is the need for nurse prescribers to become better equipped in terms of their knowledge and skills regarding medications, and the monitoring and detection of physical health problems (Nolan *et al.* 2001). Finally, patients may well expect treatment advice from junior doctors and psychiatrists and may be unsure why treatment decisions have been delegated to a nurse prescriber.

Medical liaison services

Liaison services are commonplace in all major hospitals in the UK. Common mental health problems such as depression found in general hospitals are 10 times higher than those found in community settings (Koenig & Blazer 1992). Psychiatric liaison services can have a positive effect on screening and subse-quent treatment of depression for those people who are admitted with medical problems.

One of the commonest reasons for emergency medical treatment in the UK are those people who present with self-harm. It is estimated that 170 000 cases are people who self-harm and present to UK hospitals and this is the highest in Europe (Cook 2004). Many terms have been used to describe self-harm, such as attempted suicide, intentional overdose and self-mutilation (National Collaborating Centre for Mental Health 2004). The attitudes of health professionals working in acci-dent and emergency departments may militate against engagement and positive health-promoting behaviours (NIMHE 2006). Mental health nurses with prescrip-tive authority can offer follow-up services to assess symptoms and problem-solv-ing techniques. Short-term prescribing of medication may be one of the solutions.

Hard-to-reach groups

Nurse prescribers need to think about providing interventions to people who suffer health inequalities. There are many examples such as homeless people with mental illness (Whiting 2007), people who live in – deprived housing estates, asylum and migrant workers and people who are in prison. Such disadvantaged groups tend to have poor physical health, combined with mental health problems or a learning difficulty. Access to psychiatrists or general practitioners may not always be available.

Disease and condition areas

This section will examine how nurse prescribers could work with disease areas in a range of care settings.

Dementia

Patients who are over 65 years occupy two-thirds of hospital beds (Age Concern 2008), but health services are not geared towards meeting their mental health or physical care needs (DoH 2007d). The problem is particularly acute in the UK because there are approximately 700 000 people with dementia and this will rise to 1.7 million by 2051 (Dementia UK 2007).

Dementia can be defined as a syndrome characterised as acquired cognitive deficits resulting from central neurodegenerative and ischaemic changes. Alzheimer's disease and vascular dementia are two common forms. The chronicity of the condition and its heavy toll on the carer will place strain on services to cope with demand and deliver quality care. NICE (2006a) guidelines have been developed to support professionals in the assessment and treatment of people with dementia.

It is sad that no cure exists for this tragic disorder. New types of drugs are available to slow the progression of the disease and extend the quality of the patient's life (Table 7.2). Antidementia drugs have provided pharmacological options with a new lease of life (NICE 2007a). They slow down the progression of the disorder. The aim of treatment is to improve the patient's cognition, daily living and behaviour and reduce carer burden. Problems for the sufferer and carer emerge when early diagnosis and treatment is put off by ill-informed service response.

Guidance suggests that all three acetylcholinesterase inhibitor (AChEI) drugs are efficacious and should be considered for patients if they score between 10 and 20 on the mini-mental state examination (NICE 2007a). It is essential to diagnose Alzheimer's disease as quickly as possible. In a given population of people with dementia, 50% will be diagnosed and a further 50% offered treatment. When treatment is given, for many it is curtailed before a full evaluation of the drug (Stahl 2006). The challenge in assessment is to differentiate Alzheimer's disease from other organic pathologies such as drug toxicity, infections and depressive symptoms and hence the development of a memory service clinic to screen for Alzheimer's disease.

Table 7.2 Types of drugs used to treat dementia

Type	Drug	Benefits	Side effects and disadvantages	Action
Acetylcholinesterase inhibitors (AChEI)	Donepezil	Require intact target sites for effectiveness of treatment Suitable for early-onset dementia Once-daily dosing	Gastrointestinal disturbance, for example, nausea and vomiting	Selective inhibitor of AChEI
	Galantamine	Enables cholinesterase levels to increase to promote cognition for moderate cases Once-daily dosing	Gastrointestinal disturbance, for example, nausea and vomiting	Selective inhibitor of AChEI; affects nicotinic receptors
	Rivastigmine	Enables cholinesterase levels to increase to promote cognition for moderate cases Twice-daily dosing Available as a patch	Gastrointestinal disturbance for example, nausea and vomiting Up to 29% people withdraw from treatment	Selective inhibitor of AChEI No hepatic interactions with other drugs
Neuropeptide inhibitors	Memantine	Used for moderate-to-severe cases of Alzheimer's disease	Neurological disturbance, for example, disorientation and hallucinations Not recommend as first-line treatment (NICE 2007a)	Prevent excess stimulation of the glutamate system

Nurse prescribers can be at the heart of this team supporting psychiatrists in the delivery of assessment and treatment. Nurse prescribing has been successfully implemented in dementia services (Grant *et al.* 2007; Barlow *et al.* 2008). The progression of the disorder can be stopped in just over half of people who take AChEI for a 6-month period and a quarter actually improve over this time period. The disease however is progressive and treatment may need to be stopped when mini-mental state examination scores drop below 10 if there are no benefits of staying on medication.

A nurse prescriber working in a memory clinic can also contribute to wider care planning activities such as contributing to the diagnosis of more complex pre-sentations. This may involve collecting more information on the social context of the disorder, particularly the amount of family support available.

One of the strengths of nurse prescribing is the form of discourse used by nurses to convey information. The difficult and emotional component of conveying to loved ones or patients themselves that they have Alzheimer's disease takes time. The nurse prescriber would also be involved in devising and executing care plans to support the patient at home.

Case Study

A memory clinic has been established for over 3 years and provides an assessment and treatment service for a population of 300 000. The area has a high proportion of people over the age of 65. The majority of the work (85%) that comes to the clinic is for dementia, although clinic services are available to all people with memory problems.

Sue is a nurse prescriber and has 124 patients who enter her pathway for moderate dementia. Patients who have complex social difficulties, complex comorbid physical conditions or those with an unclear diagnosis are seen by the psychiatrist. The purpose of the memory clinic is to carry out specific tests to determine cognitive function and gather relevant information for people suspected of having dementia. On the first visit to the clinic, the nurse prescriber carries out a holistic assessment. The aim is to find out the nature of the memory problem, its history and the impact of poor memory on daily functioning.

Harry presented with a 4-year history of having cerebrovascular accidents and a 5-year history of type 2 diabetes. The family reported that Harry had presented with difficulties in finding his way back from the shop when he went for his morning paper. He was also getting up in the early hours, thinking it was morning, and then wandering around the housing estate. Harry scored 14 in the mini-mental state examination. He was prescribed donepezil 5 mg per day, which was increased to 10 mg per day by the fourth week of treatment [drug used for mild to moderate dementia (BNF 2008)]. This dose was selected because of the once-daily dosing schedule and the fact that his daughter could give him the medication before he went to bed at night. Sue provided routine monitoring of the patient over 3 months and then reassessed to ensure that the benefits of medication were still being maintained.

Schizophrenia

Schizophrenia is a serious lifelong condition. In a population of 100 000, there will be 770 people with schizophrenia. There will be 18 new episodes of schizophrenia per year (NICE 2002a). Of all people who develop schizophrenia, 25% will have a chronic remitting course. Unfortunately, up to 13% of people will end their life (Meltzer & Okayli 1995). This debilitating illness presents a huge economic burden, and in 2002, its direct care costs alone accounted for over £1bn (NICE 2002a).

Schizophrenia often manifests in early adult age and is characterised by a loss of contact with reality, false perceptions, delusions and loss of executive functioning. Social functioning is often impaired, leading to loss of social status, earnings and quality of life (Andreasen & Carpenter 1993; Stahl 2003). Schizophrenia is believed to be caused by an imbalance of dopamine in the mesolimbic and mesocortical neural pathways in the brain. The role of medication is to control the dopamine imbalance. Other neurotransmitters such as serotonin and glutamate are also implicated in schizophrenia (Tamminga & Lahti 1996). Vulnerability to schizophrenia from genetic factors, lifestyle and family stress explain why some people develop schizophrenia and then go on to suffer relapse (Zubin & Spring 1977).

The efficacy of medication treatment options for people with schizophrenia is beyond question. However, what is up for debate is the range of side effects that emerge soon after starting treatment and why up to 74% of patients discontinue their medication within 18 months (Lieberman *et al.* 2005).

First-generation antipsychotic medications were first used in the 1950s, the first of which was chlorpromazine. Further drugs were created and patients' symptoms and behaviour controlled (Healy 2006). The downside, however, was the range of unacceptable side effects, the most distressing being extrapyramidal side effects. Drugs such as chlorpromazine [drug licensed for the treatment of schizophrenia (BNF 2008)] failed to treat the negative symptoms of schizophrenia (Table 7.3).

Second-generation antipsychotic medications came about in the 1990s. These drugs were able to control symptoms to the same degree of efficacy as the first-generation drugs were and became popular because of their perceived kinder side effect profile. A number of independently sponsored, large naturalistic population studies have since cast doubt on the various claims of tolerability (Lieberman *et al.* 2005). Gray *et al.* (2005) labelled the neurological and metabolic side effects of these medicines as the contemporary equivalent of the latter-day 'tardive dyskinesia' (side effect commonly seen in asylum patients). These drugs are also considerably more expensive than the first-generation drugs.

Third-generation drugs such as aripiprazole are now being marketed on the perceived weaknesses of first-generation and second-generation antipsychotic medications. Aripiprazole is a novel dopamine partial agonist in that it enhances and reduces excess dopamine in pathways associated with negative and positive symptoms of schizophrenia, respectively (Burris *et al.* 2002). The efficacy of this drug has been established, proving to have a tolerable side effect profile (Chrzanowski *et al.* 2006) (Table 7.3).

Table 7.3   Medication used to treat the symptoms of schizophrenia

Type	Drug	Benefits	Side effects	Action
First generation	Chlorpromazine	Treat positive symptoms	Weight gain Sedation Tardive dyskinesia	Dopamine 2 antagonist in striatum and pituitary gland
	Haloperidol	Gold standard for efficacy Less expensive than second-generation and third-generation drugs	Proneness to extrapyramidal side effects	Dopamine 2 antagonist in striatum, pituitary gland, mesolimbic and mesocortical pathway
Second generation	Quetiapine	Low threshold for weight gain	Postural hypotension	Dopamine 2 antagonist Serotonin 2A antagonist
	Risperidone	Off patent and so cheaper than other atypical drugs Low threshold for weight gain Treats negative symptoms	Prone to cause extrapyramidal side effects on doses above 6 mg but can occur in lower doses Elevation in prolactin, leading to possible sexual dysfunction	Dopamine 2 antagonist Alpha 2 antagonist
Third generation	Aripiprazole	Minimal weight gain Minimal rise in prolactin	Mimics extrapyramidal side effects Gastrointestinal disturbance Dizzyness, insomnia	Partial agonist at dopamine 2 receptors and 5HT1A receptors

The aim of treatment is to achieve adequate symptom control, if not remission, and to do this with minimum side effects. Not all patients respond the same to antipsychotic medication. NICE (2002b) guidance suggests that all newly diagnosed cases of schizophrenia should be offered the choice of a second-generation drug. Again, a second-generation drug should be considered when established cases of schizophrenia relapse. When patients present with a treatment-resistant form of schizophrenia, clozapine should be offered as soon as practicable (NICE 2002b).

Acute onset psychosis

Acute onset psychosis can occur as a one-off event or as part of a depressive or mood disorder. The aim of treatment is to arrive at a diagnosis, formulation and consideration given to an antipsychotic medication. This is important, given the period of untreated psychosis and longer term prognosis, particularly for those patients who have a first-onset psychosis (McGorry 2000; Perkins *et al.* 2005).

Case Study

Richard is 20 and has been picked up by the police under Section 136 of the Mental Health Act, believing that he can read people's minds, and admitted to hospital. After a few days, it became clear that he needed an antipsychotic drug to treat his worsening psychosis. Routine blood tests excluded organic pathology.

The nurse prescriber decided to develop a clinical management plan with Richard and the psychiatrist. Because this was a new presentation, a narrow clinical management plan was formulated that listed two antipsychotic drugs, aripiprazole and risperidone [drugs licensed for the treatment of schizophrenia (BNF 2008)]. The nurse prescriber offered Richard a choice between these two drugs and he opted for aripiprazole, on the basis that it did not lead to excessive weight gain or sedation. A clinical management plan was developed that would enable the nurse to increase the aripiprazole dose from 10 mg daily up to 30 mg daily.

In this case, Richard was stabilised on a dose of 10 mg. The patient did not experience any agitation and was discharged from the psychiatric unit within 3 weeks of admission. The clinical management plan was discontinued upon discharge and the patient seen in the outpatient clinic by the consultant psychiatrist within 7 days of discharge.

This scenario has demonstrated prompt assessment, diagnosis and treatment of an acute onset psychosis. The patient was started on an atypical drug and the nurse prescriber counselled the patient on likely side effects. Patients who newly present are rightly worried about their symptoms and require extensive support and information about their medication and progress. The nurse prescriber, as part of their duties to track symptoms, was in an ideal position to deliver this advice.

Chronic schizophrenia

The following case example shows the complexity of nurse prescribing for a patient admitted with a chronic relapsing episode of schizophrenia. It is important to remember that schizophrenia is incredibly complex, and as the condition worsens through relapse or poor treatment effects, negative symptoms such as social withdrawal and emotional blunting appear.

Case Study

Jim has been suffering from schizophrenia for 10 years. He is currently prescribed quetiapine 750 mg per day, but compliance with this daily dose is questionable. He is symptomatic, which has led to his admission to hospital, believing that ghosts came in through his bedroom window at night and had sex with him. The patient was seen by the psychiatrist and the nurse prescriber who identified distorted contact with reality, emotional blunting and reduced social interaction. They concluded a relapse of his schizophrenia and considered treatment options for his additional negative symptoms.

A clinical management plan was developed that included a titration of quetiapine and initiation of another antipsychotic, in this case a long-acting injection of risperidone [both drugs licensed for the treatment of schizophrenia (BNF 2008)]. Jim agreed to this, as he sometimes forgot to take his quetiapine.

The nurse prescriber assessed Jim every 2 days and reduced the quetiapine dose by 200 mg on the first day but prescribed risperidone oral at 1 mg b.i.d. at the same time. The nurse prescriber then waited for 2 days to see if there was a reaction from the prescription of risperidone oral but did not find any. The nurse prescriber then reduced the quetiapine dose down to 400 mg and increased the risperidone dose to 3 mg per day. Jim was then given a long-acting injection of risperidone consta.

The kinetics of risperidone consta dictate that the slow release of the drug occurs after 14 days, with a sudden drop down to baseline levels within a day or two; hence a steady state is not achieved until 6 weeks of administration. By day 5 the quetiapine dose was reduced to 200 mg and the risperdal oral dose increased to 4 mg. By day 8, quetiapine was discontinued and risperidone oral prescribed at 6 mg per day. Two weeks after the first administration of risperidone consta, a second dose was administered. Jim continued to suffer distressing symptoms, but by week 5 the level of conviction in his abnormal beliefs was dropping and the nurse prescriber could easily persuade him that he was 'stressed out' by his neighbours, playing loud music at night.

This scenario illustrates the complexity of switching medication. Frequent review by the nurse prescriber both in and out of hospital was required. By week 7 the patient was discharged from hospital and it was agreed that the nurse prescriber would monitor the patient at home to reduce the oral formulation of risperidone to nil and to ensure no breakthrough symptoms occurred on the long-acting injection of risperidone consta for a period of 4 weeks post discharge. Since coming out of hospital, Jim was less bothered by his worries and, most importantly, re-established contact with his friends.

Bipolar affective disorder

Bipolar affective disorder is typically a condition where a patient has episodes of mania and depression. The most common is of a depressed mood. Bipolar affective disorder can be distinguished between patients who have episodes of mania and depression and patients who have depression and hypomania. Bipolar affective disorder for some people can be recurrent and therefore its effects on everyday functioning become potentially disruptive. Suicide rate is very high in this diagnostic group, being at least 20 times higher than the general population (Tondo *et al.* 2003).

Patients diagnosed with bipolar affective disorder follow a protracted illness trajectory. They are likely to experience 8–12 depressive episodes and 4–9 manic episodes during their lifetime. The disorder is associated with dying 9 years younger and losing around 12 years of normal good health. Mortality varies from 10 to 60%. Evidence indicates a significant biological basis for bipolar affective disorder, but psychological factors are also important (Lam & Wong 1997). This calls for nurse prescribers trained in pharmacological and psychological interventions (Table 7.4).

NICE (2006c) guidelines have been developed to support prescribing advice. The prescribing algorithm for bipolar disorder is complex and requires careful review at regular intervals. For patients who enter into a manic phase and who are prescribed an antidepressant medication, this should be stopped (NICE 2006c). Nurse prescribers need to weigh up the risks of abrupt discontinuation and the risk of withdrawal states as these emerge for some antidepressants. They then need to consider prescribing one of the licensed antipsychotics such as olanzapine or aripiprazole (BNF 2008). High levels of arousal could be treated with a benzodiazepine. For patients who respond poorly to the antipsychotic

Table 7.4   Nonpharmacological interventions to be used with people who suffer from bipolar affective disorder and psychotic disorders

Intervention type	Rationale
Cognitive behavioural therapy	Can be used to reduce the risk of relapse and symptom control
Family therapy	Supporting the family and carer for a loved one and to reduce stress within the family unit
Psycho-education	Teaching patients about their illness management and identification of their relapse signature
Case management	Engagement with a care plan to support employment, vocation and financial independence

medication when first prescribed, nurse prescribers should consider augmenting with lithium or valproate (NICE 2006c).

For patients who present with a depressive episode, the best practice is to start an antidepressant medication. If the patient is already on an antidepressant medication, the nurse prescriber should consider augmenting with lithium or valproate (NICE 2006c). An antidepressant medication should be avoided, however, for patients who are depressed but are at risk of rapid cycling or who have recently recovered from a hypomanic episode.

The following vignette provides a relatively simple treatment programme for a patient with a relapsed bipolar disorder who then accepted longer term treatment maintenance.

Case Study

Alison has been admitted to hospital with an acute onset mania. She has relapsed twice through not taking her medication. On the third admission, her mania was characterised by booking herself into a local hotel and then being found shouting at the bar man. The police were called when she refused to pay her bar bill, as she believed she was the mayor's mistress.

Bill was an independent nurse prescriber who worked in the home treatment team. He was the first clinician to see Jane and arranged her admission. Because Alison was well known to the service, a diagnosis was restated as a relapse of her bipolar disorder, based on her presenting symptoms.

Alison was prescribed olanzapine 10 mg oral daily, and within 5 days, her manic symptoms subsided. Bill then discussed the merits and demerits of starting on lithium for longer term maintenance therapy [drug used for prophylaxis of bipolar disorder (BNF 2008)]. He did this by providing information on the drugs themselves and also information from the Manic Depressive Fellowship about bipolar disorder.

Alison agreed to take lithium. It was explained that a renal function and thyroid function test would need to confirm whether she was appropriate to start taking the drug. When these were complete and results returned within normal limits, Bill prescribed lithium carbonate 400 mg to be taken at night. A lithium plasma assay was then taken 5 days after starting treatment and blood assay revealed a sub-therapeutic level of lithium (0.51 mmol/l). The dose was increased to 800 mg to be taken at night. A repeat lithium level taken 7 days later was 0.69 mmol/l. No further treatment changes were advised and Alison was discharged back home and supported through the home treatment team.

The importance of long-term maintenance therapy and engagement is paramount for patients with bipolar disorder. The nurse prescriber developed a relationship with the patient, having been part of the crisis assessment period. The nurse used this relationship to bring about longer term management of the patient's dis-order. Lithium is efficacious in reducing the rate of completed suicides as well as the number of attempted suicides by people with bipolar disorder (Schou 1997).

Depression

Depression is a common mental health disorder. In a course of 1 year, up to 30% of people will suffer from depression (Ustun *et al.* 2000). Of these cases, 5% will have a moderate-to-severe depression (1 in 20) (Ustun & Chatterji 2001). Approximately, 1 in 50 people who suffer from depression will need to be admitted to hospital (NICE 2006b). Up to 15% of these people will commit suicide (Solomon *et al.* 2000). Depression occurs equally, regardless of gender, although women are twice as likely to experience mild symptoms of depression (Ustun & Chatterji 2001). The risk of developing depressive symptoms increases with age and will be felt acutely by 2020, given the growing elderly population (Moussavi *et al.* 2007).

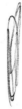

Depression can be a chronic relapsing condition. People who have suffered from a single episode of major depression are highly likely to have a repeated episode (up to 85%) (Stahl 2000). The burden of the disease impacts on the patient's social and economic mobility. It has a greater negative impact on their quality of life. Depression has a profound economic impact: 70 million work-days are lost annually because of depression (NICE 2006b).

There are guidelines that place people with depression into a stepped care arrangement (NICE 2006b). In steps 1–3, people typically present with mild-to-moderate depression and are managed in a primary care setting. Step 4 covers treatment of depression by specialist mental health services and step 5 covers inpatient treatment of depression (NICE 2006b).

Depression in its simplest form is a disturbance of mood or an exaggeration of mood from everyday occurrences that brings about sadness. Various symptoms must be present that affect the person's physical and mental well-being. The ICD-10 identifies 10 symptoms of which 4 must be present for mild depression, 6 for moderate and 8 for severe depression (Cooper 1994). The symptoms must be present for more than 2 weeks for all 3 clusters (Murray & Lopez 1996).

People with depression have an imbalance of chemicals in the brain known as neurotransmitters, particularly too little serotonin and noradrenaline activity (Ressler & Nemroff 2000). There are several drug therapies available to treat depression. These have been developed over the past 50 years.

First-generation antidepressant drugs were the tricyclic antidepressants (TCAs) and monoamine oxidase inhibitors (MAOIs) developed in the late 1950s (Cookson *et al.* 2002). TCAs block the reuptake of serotonin and noradrenaline into the presynaptic neurone (Stahl 2003). The disadvantages of TCAs are that they produce anticholinergic and antihistamineric side effects such as dry mouth, drowsiness and weight gain. These types of drugs can be potentially lethal in overdose, given their effect on the cardiac system (Wilkinson *et al.* 1990). Examples of TCAs include amitriptyline and imipramine (BNF 2008).

MAOIs increase both serotonin and noradrenaline transmission at the synapse by preventing their reuptake (Stahl 2000). MAOIs are often used as a third-line treatment for depression (NICE 2006b). The common side effects of MAOIs are postural hypotension, nausea and sexual difficulties (Taylor *et al.* 2007). A major disadvantage of MAOIs is the potential lethal interaction between certain foods that contain tyramine (e.g. cheese and bovril). Examples of MAOIs include phenelzine and tranylcypromine (BNF 2008).

Second-generation antidepressants are selective serotonin reuptake inhibitors (SSRIs). SSRIs prevent the reuptake of serotonin in the presynaptic cleft and so increase serotonin neurotransmission (Cookson *et al.* 2002). The side effects most associated with SSRIs are agitation, anxiety and sexual dysfunction (Stahl 2000). Nurse prescribers need to be cautious in prescribing SSRIs for patients who are younger than 25, given the potential for increased suicidal ideation. Examples of SSRIs include citalopram and fluoxetine (BNF 2008).

Case Study

James was admitted to hospital with a heart attack. After a few days on the ward, he had sleep disturbance and a worsening mood as the day progressed and was also ambivalent about getting well. He was referred to the psychiatric liaison nurse, Mary, who is an independent prescriber. Upon investigation, it was found that the patient had just been made redundant and his two older sons recently left home after finding employment some distance away.

Mary diagnosed depressive symptoms of moderate severity and discussed the different types of antidepressant therapy alongside nonpharmacological interventions such as cognitive behavioural therapy. In order for James to choose his treatment, Mary explained how drugs worked and what side effects were most likely. James agreed on the SSRI drug citalopram because of its reduced potential for drug-to-drug interactions. Mary prescribed an initial starting dose of citalopram 20 mg daily [drug licensed for the treatment of depression (BNF 2008)]. She explained to James that treatment response usually took 2 weeks but she would see him every 2–3 days on the medical ward. Upon investigation, Mary found that James developed a dry mouth and anxiety symptoms, which they discussed together and agreed to monitor to see if these worsened over time.

A care plan was devised that covered the prescription of medication, its effect and how progress in recovery would impact on longer term functioning when James returned home. Mary provided after-care support to him when he was discharged from hospital and reviewed treatment every 2 weeks until 12 weeks had elapsed. James was then discharged from the liaison service back to the care of the general practitioner.

Nonpharmacological interventions are important considerations for people who suffer from depression (Layard 2006). Nurse prescribers should be trained to deliver psychological therapies in a combined fashion if required. Evidence suggests that patients and doctors may have differences in opinion on what best suits patients' need in terms of treatment option (Bedi *et al.* 2000). The key message is that patients should be offered a choice. For this, patients need to be involved in the decision-making process about what would work best for them if the chances of remaining with treatment are to be successful (Loh *et al.* 2007). The role of the liaison nurse here underscores the importance of diagnosing conditions such as depression when they copresent with acute medical conditions.

The independent prescriber, in this instance, was able to build a collaborative relationship with the patient and longer term concordance when he left hospital.

Nicotine addiction

There is a huge public health agenda to help people quit smoking. People who enter hospital and smoke could be targeted for their willingness to stop smoking and to take advantage of the 'teachable moment' (Rigotti *et al.* 2007). The teachable moment can also occur when patients are assessed at home by their community psychiatric nurse. NICE (2006d, 2007a, 2008) has issued guidelines on the types of drugs used to treat nicotine addiction and the best ways for nurses to target people who smoke. Nicotine replacement therapy is the first-line choice of treatment (NICE 2002c) although there are alternatives based on the patients presentation (Table 7.6).

There are a number of relevant areas for nurses to consider before prescribing medication for nicotine addiction (Table 7.5). Nurses need to see smoking cessation as a programme of long-term intervention that combines pharmacological and behavioural interventions (Jones & Jones 2008).

Although the patient did not completely abstain from smoking, he passed a further quit attempt and this can be used as a positive experience further along the treatment trajectory.

Table 7.5   Factors to consider when assessing readiness for smoking cessation

Nicotine intake, for how long and how many quit attempts

Interaction between nicotine and prescribed medication

Metabolism of drugs

Health expectations

Use of nicotine to control symptoms

Table 7.6   Types of drugs to be used in smoking cessation

Type	Drug	Consideration	Types
Nicotine replacement therapy	Nicotine	Cardiovascular disease	Nicotine gum, patches, nasal spray, inhalers, lozenges
Selective nicotine partial agonist	Varenicline	Not to be used with people under 18 or those who are breastfeeding	Tablets
	Bupropion	Not to be used with patients with a history of seizure; need to give consideration when used with antipsychotic medication	Tablets

Case Study

Ken is seen by Jen, an independent prescriber who works in alcohol services. Ken has stated that he wishes to give up smoking. Jen takes an in-depth smoking history and finds out that Ken has tried to quit six times previously. Ken has tried nicotine replacement patches but kept on forgetting to use them in the right order. For example, he would replace them after 2 days and then end up using his supply of patches.

As part of the prescribing process, Jen discussed a number of factors such as the effects and side effects of medication, the range of products and delivery mechanisms. Ken expressed his preference for varenicline so that his cravings would be reduced and Jen agreed to prescribe it as part of his abstinent-contingent treatment plan [drug licensed to aid smoking cessation (BNF 2008)]. Ken agreed to stop smoking on an agreed quit date. This is important because varenicline needs to be prescribed 2 weeks before the quit date.

Jen prescribed varenicline at a dose of 500 mcg once daily for 3 days and then 500 mcg b.i.d. for 4 days. A further dose titration was made by prescribing the drug at 1 mg for 11 days. Jen also plugged Ken into the local smoking cessation service that was being run in the local community centre.

Ken's difficulties in using previous treatments necessitated regular review of his treatment. Jen used the visits to reinforce the motivational work being completed by the cessation service. Ken went on to abstain from smoking from his quit date for 7 weeks but then started to smoke again.

Insomnia

A common symptom that crosses all areas of mental health is insomnia. Normal sleep is subjective, but generally, adults sleep between 7 and 8 h per night (Benson 2006). Common sleep disorders arise in older people when breathing stops during sleep because of airway blockage. Up to 15% of the population suffer from restless leg syndrome, a common cause of sleep disturbance. This is commonly characterised by an urge to move one's legs (Zucconi & Ferini-Strambi 2004).

There are many factors that trigger periods of poor sleep that then develop into insomnia. These range from lifestyle factors such as excessive caffeine and nicotine intake. Depression, anxiety and dementia are common conditions that feature in insomnia. Particularly in older people, insomnia is both caused by and worsened by coexisting medical conditions.

Insomnia and its treatment should not be approached lightly as the historical legacy of tolerance and dependence was a major problem for the older hypnotic drugs. Quite probable is the misdiagnosis of insomnia. In a large review of epidemiological data, up to 48% of people experienced difficulty in sleeping but only 6% were able to meet the diagnostic criteria for insomnia (NICE 2004a).

The need for augmentation with sleep hygiene interventions is a requirement here for nurse prescribers. As an understanding and application of cognitive behavioural therapy techniques, relaxation therapy could also be used where patients show a resistive form of insomnia (Table 7.7).

The types of drugs used to treat insomnia should be based on evidence-based guidelines and nurse prescribers should ensure that patients who fall outside the guidelines be passed on to more knowledgeable practitioners (Table 7.8).

Table 7.7   Nonpharmacological considerations to promote sleep hygiene

Factor	Intervention	Rationale
Diet	Limit caffeinated drinks to 2 units per day before lunch time Limit alcohol to 1 unit per day Light protein-based bedtime snack such as milk	Caffeine blocks adenosine receptors and thus stimulates the brain Alcohol has a short half-life and withdrawal occurs late at night Reduces hypoglycaemia
Environment	Increase sun exposure during the day and reduces light content during the night If unable to sleep after 30 min, get up and leave the bedroom Engage in relaxing activity until need to sleep arrives	The human body has circadian rhythms regulated by natural light and darkness Cognitive association between bedroom and restful activities
Functioning	Active physical activity during the day Avoid passive activity such as watching TV	Higher levels of functioning during daylight hours prevent napping Association between relaxing activities such as sleep

Table 7.8   Commonly used drugs for the treatment of insomnia

Type	Drug	Benefits	Side effects	Action
Nonbenzodiazepine hypnotic	Zopiclone Zolpidem	Slower action but longer lasting for the three Z-drugs Less chance of dependence Can be prescribed by an independent prescriber Rapid acting (within 15 min)	Daytime sedation Ataxia Diarrhoea Memory disturbance	Selective binding to benzodiazepine receptor Increases GABA inhibitory responses Binds to omega 1 benzodiazepine receptor
Benzodiazepine hypnotic	Temazepam	Helpful to reverse night-time wakening	Daytime sedation	Binds to benzodiazepine receptors
This is a controlled drug and so only prescribed by supplementary prescribers			Dependence forming	Increases effects of GABA

The evidence base supporting nonpharmacological interventions is growing, particularly around activities or lifestyle behaviour that stimulates parts of the brain or disrupts 24-h circadian rhythms.

For adults, a nonbenzodiazapine drug, commonly called the Z-drugs, should be prescribed for up to 10 days (NICE 2004a). Current NICE (2004a) guidance suggests no clinically significant difference between the three Z-drugs and the shorter acting benzodiazepine hypnotic drugs. The rationale for prescribing may therefore be considered against the costs and the choices expressed by patients as and when they experience the drug.

The following vignette will go through the process for diagnosing the problem of insomnia.

Case Study

Jane works as an advanced nurse practitioner in a primary care polyclinic in a busy inner-city locality. Jim comes to see her, complaining of an inability to sleep and then stay asleep. Jane carries out a physical examination and then proceeds to a sleep assessment, specifically the duration and pattern of night-time sleep. Use of alcohol and over-the-counter medication was subsequently screened. The main intervention was to teach sleep hygiene techniques and to gather monitoring data.

Jane provided education on promoting sleep hygiene, which included learning to wake up at the same time each day and to resist the temptation to sleep during the day. It was important for Jim to do a short exercise such as a walk during the morning and, as the day progressed, to avoid heavy exercise late at night. An important environmental change is to make sure the bedroom stays cooler than the rest of the house by turning down the radiator in the room. Jim was asked to maintain a sleep diary for the next 3 nights and return to the clinic.

After 3 days, Jim reported sleep maintenance insomnia. Jane decided to prescribe the nonbenzodiazepine receptor agonist, zopiclone, at 7.5 mg for 7 nights and asked Jim to return the following week for review [drug licensed for the treatment of insomnia (BNF 2008)]. Evidence to support this choice of drug is that zopiclone is better at maintaining the architecture of sleep (Dundar *et al.* 2004). Jane advised Jim to refrain from taking alcohol even when he started to feel better with improved sleep. Jim was informed that he might experience residual sleepiness during the day and headaches.

As this vignette has demonstrated, the independent prescriber diagnosed the problem by enquiring about the patient's sleep architecture. Areas covered included the person's view on their sleep pattern, latency, duration, sleep disturbances, and any use of prescribed or over-the-counter medications. It is important to note the amount of daytime lethargy and napping, as this can be particularly troublesome to promote sleep. The actions taken by the independent prescriber included both pharmacological and nonpharmacological interventions because, in reality, a sole approach is limited.

The golden rule with diagnosis and treatment of insomnia is to reserve pharmacological interventions until nonpharmacological interventions have been exhausted. The prescription of certain psychotropic medication to promote sleep can go on to cause their own problems, particularly for older people.

Opioid addiction

There is a national shortage of addiction psychiatrists (Hoadley *et al.* 2005). Changes to the Misuse of Drugs Regulations (Home Office 2001) have enabled nurse prescribers to prescribe controlled substances. This amended piece of legislation transformed the stranglehold on who could prescribe controlled substances (Barcroft 2005). This problem is compounded by general practitioner prescribing that is ill informed of the wider substance misuse agenda. Prior to the amendment and even now, nurses working in addiction services provide guidance on how best to prescribe medication. The problems encountered for addiction services are long waiting times for treatment. Examples of innovative services where nurse prescribers can feature in the prescribing of controlled drugs such as methadone are emerging (Gallagher *et al.* 2006; Harniman 2007).

Methadone and buprenorphine are licensed for the treatment and prevention of opioid dependence, with methadone being recommended as the first-line choice of treatment (NICE 2007b). NICE (2007b) issued guidelines setting out how methadone should be used. An optimal dose of methadone is achieved usually over a 4-week period. Very close attention is required when initiating methadone treatment within the first 2 weeks to avoid its toxicity. The starting dose of methadone is between 10 and 30 mg per day and, following the first week, can be increased again up to 60–120 mg per week, although the dose increments need to be spaced out over a number of weeks.

The principles of prescribing methadone are to prescribe an effective dose that minimises cravings for heroin and then to minimise the risk of overdose. Risk factors identified for overdose on methadone include patients having a low tolerance for opioids, patients taking alcohol along with methadone and the prescription of too high an initial dose. Nurses need to be aware that toxicity is cumulative and builds up over several days of treatment. This is because methadone has a long half-life and may be up to 50 h for people who have a chronic drug problem (National Treatment Agency 2007).

Case Study

Julie is a nurse consultant in substance misuse and a supplementary nurse prescriber. Julie has been working with Jake for 2 months regarding attempts to control the use of heroin. Priorities in these first few weeks have been to minimise the sharing of needles with other users. Jake turns up at the team base in a heightened state of arousal. He has not used heroin for 12 h and is starting to withdraw. He has beads of sweat on his forehead and a tachycardia of 98 beats per minute.

Julie has taken a detailed history of drug misuse, including duration of use, quantity and route of administration. A diagnosis of opioid dependence was reconfirmed. Julie has previously undertaken an assessment of prescribing methadone and Jake was now ready to give this treatment a chance to work [drug licensed for opioid dependence (BNF 2008)].

Jake was taking a £10 bag of heroin daily. Julie prescribed 20 mg of methadone as the first daily dose. Jake stayed in the clinic to see if the treatment effect was achieved, and after half an hour, his withdrawal symptoms improved. Julie then asked him to return to the clinic every day at 10 AM to receive his supervised administration and also to review longer term tolerance.

Given that steady state takes approximately 5 days, Julie went on to prescribe a further 10 mg daily dose on day 8. Further daily supervised administration doses were transferred to the local pharmacy.

After 6 weeks of 30 mg per day of methadone, Jake was on a stable dose. He was not using heroin but was taking 20 units of alcohol per week. This information became apparent only when Julie visited Jake at home and found empty tins of normal strength lager in his refuge bin outside his door. However, on the up side, Jake was engaged in methadone maintenance, was not using heroin and was seeing his drug worker on a weekly basis.

Drug treatment engagement outcomes are better for people when they have a consistent relationship with their prescriber (Meier *et al.* 2005). There are potentially more nurses who can prescribe controlled substances than there are psychiatrists, so nurses would be in a better position to maximise the tactics of stable engagement over a long period of time.

Benefits realisation from this way of working led to increased frequency of review of medication and less delay in carrying out the review. The vignette also demonstrates a different way to build relationships with patients. Difficulties with this model of working may be where patients have chaotic drug misuse or where they are transferred between treatment settings. The realities of substance misuse are that all patients are not suitable for nurse prescribing.

Conclusion

This chapter has helped to bring to life situations where nurse prescribing can be used and the different types of nurse prescribing. The process of prescribing medication is a complex activity. It requires advanced skills to perform an examination, formulate treatment and evaluate the outcome of that treatment.

The vignettes illustrate the variation in prescribing in mental health. The vastness of the area demonstrates the importance of not straying from your clinical competencies without supervision. This is not to say that nurses cannot learn about the use of other drugs for conditions that sit alongside their area. It requires careful dissection of what learning is required and how competencies will be assessed.

The range of services where nurses can prescribe medication is limited by the mindset of the organisation. Nurses with the correct skill set can provide prescriptive intervention to bring benefits for patient care. There are services that are aligned with mental health but are not covered in this chapter, not because they are not suitable, rather because of the limitations of space in the book.

Chapter 8
Promoting concordance and patient involvement in medication management

Introduction

In the Audit Commission's report 'A spoonful of sugar' (2001) and later in 'Medicines management: everybody's business' (DoH 2007b), the authors define medicines management as 'the entire way that medicines are selected, procured, delivered, prescribed, administered and reviewed to optimise the contribution that medicines make to producing desired outcomes of patient care'. The reality of patients being active partners in the type of medication prescribed with an explanation of how it works may be somewhat different.

This chapter will cover the main types of intervention to support patients to take medication. The use of case examples will illustrate clinical issues for consideration by a nurse prescriber in their endeavours to support patients to take medication. It is important to remember that no one strategy is correct for all types of patient. The main point of this chapter is to help nurses understand and apply the principles of involving patients in deciding about their health and treatment.

What is concordance?

Health care professionals use the terms concordance, adherence and compliance almost as though they are interchangeable. The terms compliance and adherence are somewhat different as they reflect the situation where the nurse prescriber would be persuading the patient to take their medication. Concordance can be defined as where the prescriber would work with the patient and discuss their beliefs about medication and how they would wish to take medication in a shared partnership (Blenkinsopp et al. 1997). To satisfy this definition, nurses would need to have and demonstrate competencies in expert interpersonal skills such as listening to patients, helping patients to understand their illness and what treatment works best and checking for understanding regarding the information we give to people (Latter 2005).

When one looks at concordance, it seems as although there is still a power differential within the relationship because it would still be the nurse prescriber who would decide prescribing a particular medication. Some patients may prefer not to take medication and this may be an agreed outcome from the consultation. Advancement from concordance is the aspect of choice. This is where patients would be offered choices in the range of medicines that are put before them.

The nurse prescriber would not have any real value placed on the medicinal products and their only intention would be to stay within the categories for which the drugs are prescribed.

It is important for the nurse prescriber to adopt a value base that respects the beliefs and wishes of the patients (National Prescribing Centre 2007). Fundamental to this value base is the recognition that the patient is an equal partner within the prescribing relationship (Jones & Jones 2007a,b). However, the question arises that how equal is the patient. The prescriber has an in-depth knowledge of signs, symptoms, treatment efficacy and outcomes built up through clinical experience and education. The patient has a 'lived experience' source of knowledge about their illness. They may be aware of their symptoms and what relief they can expect from nonpharmacological techniques. More so, their lifestyle can affect their symptoms. There are some situations where patients may have limited insight into their symptoms and do not recognise the language used by health professionals to describe their experiences.

On the other hand, some patients are accustomed to a didactic approach where they simply comply with the health intervention. This is where the problems of compliance therapy fall down. It was assumed that all patients could somehow be manipulated or cajoled to take their medicines.

Why does poor concordance matter?

The amount of psychiatric medication prescribed accounts for about 3% of overall budget of an NHS trust and 16% of nonpay expenditure. On psychiatric units, 91% of patients take two or more medications for their psychiatric and coexisting medical problems (Healthcare Commission 2006, 2007a,b). Poor compliance with medication is a costly endeavour to NHS resource because ultimately the medication is discarded and wasted. Certain types of psychiatric medication are very expensive and ways must be found to lessen the amount of these medicines from going waste.

Patients with mental health problems have concerns about taking medication (Gray *et al.* 2005). Very often, treatment options are not discussed with them and little information is given to them about the medication. These findings were echoed by two independent reviews examining the quality of prescribing in mental health services (NPSA 2006, Healthcare Commission 2007a). Patients also choose not to take medication because of perceived poor control over their residual symptoms and their desire to use other techniques.

A large body of evidence points towards a problem in ensuring that people with psychotic conditions take their medication. In the case of people with schizophrenia, 74% of patients discontinue their medication within 18 months of its first prescription (Lieberman *et al.* 2005). For people with schizophrenia, discontinuation from medication can lead to relapse in their condition and rehospitalisation (NICE 2002b).

When mental health patients relapse on a number of occasions, their overall level of functioning deteriorates, resulting in longer hospital stays and shorter periods between the relapse episodes (Helgason 1990). In the second UK report on suicides and homicides in people with mental health problems, clinicians identified that noncompliance with medication was associated with an increased risk factor for violent behaviour (Appleby 2006).

It is important for people to take their medication for a whole range of reasons. When patients stop taking their medication, they may become ill and so be unable to work. Loss of meaningful activity through occupation is associated with social breakdown, family fragmentation and an economic deficit to the country as a whole. When patients relapse, the burden of care is picked up by family members, thus leading to potential for carer burnout that then leads to problems for the carer in terms of their own physical and mental health. Loss of family support would also aggravate a further deterioration in the patient's condition. The overall family and social disruption through noncompliance becomes a major driver to address this issue.

Why people stop taking medication?

Patients may stop taking their medication for very simple reasons. They may not have the same level of understanding about their illness or the need for medication compared to the prescriber. Providing patients with information about their medication is a crucial step in gaining their agreement. Patients also need to make a cognitive appraisal that taking the medication will do them good or the risks of not taking the medication doing them harm.

However, we have all come across clinical situations that provide plenty of reasons why our patients choose not to take their medication.

(1) Patients will act in accordance with their own personal understanding of the choices that are laid before them, that is a health belief model.
(2) Patients who feel in control of their destiny and who believe they can administer their own medication or have choices about how they take their medication will more likely comply with treatment.
(3) Patients that come from different cultures. An example would be prescribing an antipsychotic medication to a patient who comes from a culture where people believe in witchcraft. Problems would arise when the nurse would not spend time with the patient and the carer to distinguish between cultural beliefs about witchcraft and the features of psychosis that are evident at clinical examination.
(4) Some patients may unintentionally forget to take medication because of the poor quality of the advice given to them during consultation.
(5) There are some simple practical reasons also. Some patients receive prescriptions but do not take them to the pharmacy.

A standard medical textbook method of communicating to patients the product of a diagnostic decision and treatment plan usually follows a number of steps. It is explained to the patient why a particular medication has been chosen. The dosing schedule is given, and also the likely effects and side effects of the medication

(Gelder *et al.* 2004). Patients would naturally want to find out how long it takes medication to work and how long they should take the drug for. Some patients leave the consultation with an unclear understanding about their medication and then suffer further degradation in knowledge and understanding as time goes on.

Strategies to help people take their medication

Effective prescribing has been studied and general guidance offered to help nurse prescribers develop their competency (National Prescribing Centre 2007). Two major aspects are the relationship developed with the patient and the core values held by the nurse in terms of medicines management.

Compliance research in the 1970s right up to the 1990s was about finding out what prescribers needed to do to predict why a patient would be noncompliant with their medication and further to identify interventions that then went on to promote compliance. It was very much about ensuring patients take their medication and, as we have already discussed, using the professional dominance and knowledge and power held by the prescriber, and using this to best effect on the passive recipient of this information. Awareness of this problem was arrived at by a Cochrane review carried out by Haynes *et al.* (1996) where their conclusions quite rightly identified that to help patients take their medication, the prescriber would need to embrace a multimodal approach that incorporates understanding patients cognitive impressions of medication and practical strategies to help patients to remember to take their medication.

Research has been dominated by understanding the cognitive elements of non-compliance that it has led to a large multisite research trial. The study by Gray *et al.* (2006) has demonstrated that adherence therapy is no more effective in bringing about medication adherence than supporting interventions and it again casts doubt over the power relationship swayed towards the prescriber. The finding supports the need to radically change our conception of concordance to one where patients choose and are helped to choose the medication that best meets their treatment needs. The important point is for nurse prescribers to approach the encounter and treat patients as although they were individuals, and to understand the individual's appraisal of how they understand their illness and treatment.

The point has been made that simply telling patients to take their medication is ineffective. The dominance of power within the relationship has not produced better medicines management.

As part of the prescribing assessment, nurses will need to consider whether patients would intentionally forget to take their medication or whether there is a cognitive or behavioural solution to be found. Unintentional behaviour may be where patients forget or are unable to manage or understand the treatment options put before them.

Nurses need to consider concordance in all their interactions. It is well known that clinicians tend to overestimate the amount of time they invest in involving patients about the treatment nurses wish them to take (Makoul *et al.* 1995). This is why nurses need to be continually subject to awareness training about concordance and the importance of involving patients.

One must be honest with patients when they say they are concerned about the physical disorders that arise when taking psychiatric medication. Patients are distressed by the increased chances of developing metabolic disorders or having extrapyramidal side effects commonly seen as movement disorders. Extrapyramidal side effects are unpleasant to patients and at worst can lead them to take their own lives. This will require a change in consultation style as invariably prescribers would resist from such a discussion in the belief that patients would not take their medication. Patients are concerned about the efficacy of medication whilst prescribers are concerned with side effects (Gray *et al.* 2007).

What then lies at the root of helping patients to take their medication? Communication between the nurse and the patient is important. The aim is to promote stronger therapeutic engagement to bring about better understanding for patients about the medication they take. Nurses need to find out what information they require about medicines and to check how much they know already (Rollnick *et al.* 2000). A key intervention for nurses is to help patients understand side effects and what control they have over them. Generally, patients will be more receptive to information that is free from medical jargon or relayed in a fashion that leaves the patient feeling vulnerable and insecure in being able to understand the information. However, nurses must not shy away from discussing technical information about medication.

Nurses tend to forget to ask patients if they are indeed taking medication. They assume that patients do. Patients, when confronted with not taking their medication, may sometimes admit to secreting it away. Interventions to detect and support patients to take their medication are often missing. Nurse prescribers are in a unique position to influence this problem.

However it is easy for the qualities mentioned above to be mere sound bites. The fruits of nurse prescribing would best be delivered by teaching nurses to understand their own feelings and thoughts about why patients should take medication. If we do not do this, we may find that we replicate some of the problems with medical prescribing where patients perceive the doctor as the sole owner of information regarding treatment. It is notable that greater emphasis is being placed on patients as partners in their care and this has been aptly demonstrated by the expert patient programmes where patients are being taught to be active partners in the management of their long-term condition.

There is a growing evidence base on the science behind interventions to support people to take medication.

The interventions can broadly be split into:

(1) psycho education;
(2) behavioural interventions;
(3) cognitive behavioural interventions;
(4) motivational interviewing;
(5) compliance therapy.

Psycho education

This intervention is where you give the patient information about their disorder and how treatment will help them to cope with it. In order for patients to understand the reasons why they need to take medication, nurse prescribers require highly developed communication skills. It is worthwhile to remember that nurses have a duty to ensure patients understand why they should take medication before they prescribe it to them.

The intervention is geared towards giving the patient information on the medicinal product. This aspect can be split into a number of domains (Box 8.1). The process would involve a didactic process of the clinician meeting with the patient to find out deficits in knowledge and then filling in the gaps in knowledge.

Box 8.1

Use of the drug	How long to take the drug
Time before treatment	Dose range
How to take the drug	Side effects of treatment

Some patients may benefit from a group work approach. A Cochrane review of 10 studies examining psycho education reveals that providing written information and verbal information within a programme of individual sessions appears to be the essential ingredient (Pekkala & Merinder 2002). This means that people must be given more than just information. A clinical programme to ground the information must be in place.

Case Study

John is a 22-year-old man who has a diagnosis of schizophrenia. He has been in hospital for the last 5 weeks. He is showing signs of difficulty in understanding the link between taking medication and being well. John is not averse to taking medication, but the past two admissions have been precipitated in part by not taking medication.

John is invited to attend a group run by the nurse in charge of the ward, which aims to give people information about their illness and the importance of medication. The group runs for 10 sessions. Each session covers a different aspect of helping patients to take medication.

John attends 6 of the 10 sessions. He demonstrates an increased awareness of his illness and is able to describe his symptoms as voices that trouble him. John associates control over his illness with the importance of taking medication.

Behavioural interventions

The whole point of behavioural interventions is to shape, mould and change patient behaviours around taking medication. This type of intervention may be suited to patients who have unintentional problems with medication compliance. Interventions have been put forward that add in or change behaviours such as rehearsing, modelling, and changing the packaging of the medication, such as 'Venalink'. In other words, this is the change in the behaviour routine of the patient so that it aids them to take medication. A number of studies have shown improved adherence for people with schizophrenia in taking medication following the intervention. For example, Cramer & Rosenheck (1999) demonstrated the behavioural approach using simple techniques such as having special caps on pill bottles with date and time. Behavioural approach may also include using the family or carer in the behavioural prompts or the family member reminding the patient to take their medication at a set time.

Case Study

Jane is a 35-year-old depressed lady who has mild learning difficulties. Jane lives with both her parents in a three-bedroom detached property. Jane attends a day care facility for 3 days a week and this helps to support her with functional activity and social outlet. The problem is that her parents who are both elderly and frail are feeling less confident in administering Jane her daily dose of escitalopram [drug licensed for the treatment of depression (BNF 2008)]. The parents have asked the nurse to help them teach Jane about the routine of taking medication.

The nurse carries out an assessment and concludes that Jane is not opposed to taking medication but would have difficulties remembering when to take it. The problem appears to be lack of prompts in Jane's daily routine. The nurse decides to devise a behaviour-orientated care plan that helps Jane to put in place triggers and then react to those triggers leading to compliance with medication.

The nurse agrees with Jane to put a permanent note on the refrigerator to remember to take her medication. The nurse also arranges to have the medication dispensed by the pharmacy in a daily-ordered pillbox. Each day of the week is clearly labelled.

Depressed patients who are in hospital can also be encouraged to undertake activity scheduling (Tompkins 2004). This is where the nurse prescriber can encourage patients to record daily activities that bring pleasure and distress. Patients can then build in activities that provide more pleasure to their life and leads to a greater sense of self-esteem and social engagement. Activity scheduling can also increase the amount of activity patients may undertake, and this could include daytime exercise and exposure to sunlight.

Cognitive behavioural interventions

This set of interventions appears to be a mixture of giving education and crucially helping the patient to appraise the cognitive beliefs about taking the medication backed up with behavioural interventions (Gray *et al.* 2002,

Haddock *et al.* 2003)). Innovative computerised modalities have been designed (Carroll *et al.* 2008). There is evidence that a cognitive approach works in terms of reducing time that patients spend in hospital (Lecompte & Pelc 1996), control over positive symptoms of schizophrenia (Jones *et al.* 2004) and longer periods of abstinence for substance misuse (Carroll *et al.* 2008).

Evidence to support group cognitive behavioural therapy is less clear but the approach does have an effect in lowering social anxiety for people with schizophrenia (Lawrence *et al.* 2006). Evidence also supports giving people with residual depression a trial of cognitive therapy, particularly around increasing social functioning (Scott *et al.* 2000). Some argue that cognitive interventions should be focused on the symptom rather than the illness itself (Chadwick *et al.* 1996). An example is of hearing voices; in this case, the patient should be asked to grade the unpleasant feelings before and after taking medication.

A strategy that has been found helpful is to ask patients to do a benefit analysis of their decision about taking medication or not. For example, patients with schizophrenia state that they do not want to take oral medication. Try and encourage patients to think about the advantages and disadvantages of not taking medication. With this approach, it enables patients and nurse prescribers to discuss reasons why patients view medication in the way they do.

Advantages of taking oral medication	**Advantages of not taking oral medication**
Medication helps to keep me out of hospital.	I am free of popping pills.
My family are less worried.	I feel less tired throughout the day
I am able to work.	I feel normal, like other people.
Some types of medication help me.	
Disadvantages of taking oral medication	**Disadvantages of not taking oral medication**
I have to take them every day.	I have been ill before and I may get ill again.
It makes me feel tired.	Many times I have been ill and have been put in hospital.
Sometimes I feel sick.	I have joined a job in a company recently and if I get ill I may not be able to work there again.
I think medication actually harms my body.	
I tend to put on weight.	

Motivational interviewing

Motivational interviewing is a person-centred talking therapy where a clinician talks with patients about the advantages and disadvantages of taking medication.

An important step is to determine whether the patient is at a precontemplative stage about change, as this will determine the intervention (Miller & Rollnick 2004). It is not the role of the clinician to force a particular view on the patient; for example, the merits of taking medication. On the contrary, it is for the patient to choose a particular view for themselves. A good example to illustrate motivational work is substance misuse. Motivational interviewing has clinical application for people who take drugs (Baker *et al.* 2001).

Case Study

Jack is 31 and he has been using heroin intravenously for 5 years. He usually spends between £15 and £20 a day and he usually scores by using a regular dealer.

Jack has been referred to the drug service by his general practitioner. Jack has also been engaged with drug services a few times before but he has never lasted more than a few weeks of contact visits. He is aware of methadone as a substitute drug.

Julie is a substance abuse nurse consultant. Julie is aware that Jack should be offered choices in whether he wants to manage his substance misuse. Julie agrees to meet with Jack in the team office and then leads him through a process of identifying the pros and cons of using substances such as methadone as a substitute.

Jack agrees that heroin is harmful and can lead to infection with blood-borne viruses through shared needles. However, he does not want to attend the needle exchange because of the stigma. Julie continues to work with Jack to discuss the positive reasons for taking a substitute drug.

Compliance therapy

A more sophisticated development from motivational interviewing is compliance therapy, this is a combined strategy with the cognitive behavioural approach described above (Kemp *et al.* 1996). This is where a clinician engages with a discussion about the pros and cons of taking medication and a questioning of the difference between the behaviour and actions of not taking medication and what the patient says. For example, patients identify that they want to take medication so that they can stay out of hospital but then relapse because they fail to take medication and so end up back in hospital. O'Donnell *et al.* (2003) found that before therapy starts, people with a negative attitude at the start of the therapy are less likely to adhere to treatment post therapy.

It is important that nurse prescribers enable patients to discuss their illness and how it affects them in their everyday life and what they feel about taking treatment to modify their symptoms. Nurse prescribers may find it helpful to ask patients to rate the extent to which they believe they have an illness and the extent to which they can manage their illness without medication. It is important to consider what happens to their symptoms when they take medication. Asking patients to rate symptoms gives them a concrete figure and helps patients to deal with less abstract concepts such as health, illness and disease.

Nurse prescribers may wish to explore with the patient the times when they have been noncompliant with their medication and to establish if there is any pattern. For example, some patients may stop taking their medication when they feel that their symptoms have resolved. Again it may be helpful to ask patients what it has been like when they are at their optimum in terms of their symptoms. Likewise, some patients may stop taking their medication when they are still symptomatic and when they still experience the distress related to their symptoms and have little faith in their medication.

Many patients that we interview offer negative opinions about their medication. For example, some patients believe medication will make them sedated and so they simply do not take it. Rather than making rash changes, it may be better to test out the patients' assumption and to be frank with them that other alternatives could be selected if they do indeed feel sedated by their medication.

Helping vulnerable patients to take their medication

Patients who are elderly or have disabilities may be even more prone to not taking their medication as prescribed. Many older and frail people find the standard containers difficult to use.

The nurse prescriber could consider home delivery of the medication, particularly for people with learning difficulties who may have difficulties in leaving the home or in their orientation outside of the home. The nurse prescriber may also wish to consider compliance aids (e.g. dose boxes), which may be filled by the patient, the relative or the carer. Behavioural interventions could sit alongside the compliance aids. However, as we have stated before, nurse prescribers need to be aware that interventions need to be geared to the individual and not all patients can manage compliance aids, and nor are all drugs and dosages are suitable. The key message here is that compliance aids only work if the patient is unintentionally noncompliant.

There are notable issues for people who are elderly. The first amongst these is cost. Prescribing for older people is vast within the primary care setting (McGraw & Drennan 2001). It is important that the nurse prescriber is able to select an intervention to meet the needs of older people. For example, the nurse may need to look at what specific information is required for the older person and how that information can be understood to help them take their medication (Ryan & Chambers 2000). Moreover, care for older people takes place in the person's home and so adaptations to bring about compliance need to make use of prompts that arise in the patient's home.

Case Study

Ken has been an old-age community nurse for 9 years and a supplementary prescriber for 2 years. He has been a case manager for John for the last 12 months. John has dementia and is prescribed Aricept [licensed for the treatment of dementia (BNF 2008)] and citalopram [licensed for the treatment of depression (BNF 2008)] as part of the clinical management plan.

Ken is aware of the complexities of prescribing medication for the elderly. The clinical management plan is straightforward for the prescription of Aricept. Ken goes through simple steps to make sure the medication regimen helps to bring about compliance.

Firstly, he checked that all the medication prescribed for John was appropriate. He then made sure that the prescribing regimen was as simple as possible so that John could remember how to take his medication. Ken was aware that the extent of dementia was affecting John's ability to remember to take the medication at the right times. Ken arranged for John to have a memory aid inserted on the refrigerator door reminding John to take his medication. Ken had also arranged for the writing on the prescription bottle to be made larger and had tested this out by asking John to read the instructions out to him. John was moderately arthritic, so Ken had arranged for the bottles of his medication to be fitted with a device to help him open the bottles.

Attitudes about certain types of medication

At times nurses have incomplete and false impressions of medication and this limits their role in supporting patients in giving them information on how best to take the drug (Byrne *et al.* 2005). It is important for nurse prescribers to understand what their own attitudes and beliefs are about taking medication. Day *et al.* (2005a) examined the attitudes towards treatment versus the relationship with the prescriber. A strained relationship with the prescribed was predictive of negative attitude about medication. Hamann *et al.* (2004) found that the age of the psychiatrist predicted the choice of antipsychotic drug above all other factors.

Another factor is what nurses think about medication. For example, if nurses are worried about weight gain, would they take olanzapine if they developed a psychotic illness? If nurses would be unwilling to take a particular medication what affect does this have on patients. Many nurses would be thinking about long-term efficacy effect and the likelihood of the patient agreeing to have the medication administered by the community psychiatric nurse. Nurse prescribers will also be thinking about how tolerable the drug will be for patients. The following discussion will centre on the role of injections as this has evoked a range of emotions and viewpoints by mental health nurses.

Depot medication first started in the 1960s and became a frequent treatment strategy for when patients left the asylum. Older depot medication [such as flupenthixol and pipothiazine licensed for schizophrenia (BNF 2008)] has since been superseded by newer agents [such as risperidone long acting injection licensed for schizophrenia (BNF 2008)]. The older agents are associated with unpleasant neurological and metabolic side effects. Newer agents, for example risperidone long-acting injection, offer benefits over the other depot medications in that it has fewer tendencies to cause extrapyramidal side effects (BNF 2008).

Evidence shows that the typical depot medication is able to reduce the rate at which people relapse compared to the oral formulation (Babiker 1986). Unlike oral medication, where daily consumption is required to prevent relapse, the slower elimination may allow the patient to default on receiving their depot without necessarily progressing to a relapse. The nurse prescriber can ask the community nurse to visit the patient and offer them the opportunity to take the depot again.

Nurses and doctors hold particular views about medication based on their perceptions of either administering or prescribing them (Walburn *et al.* 2001). For example, there is a view that nurses believe depot injections to be painful and that patients should not be subjected to this awful experience. Some research has found that nurses believe depot medication to be an oppressive intervention and therefore damaging to the nurse–patient relationship. This view surprisingly is in contrast to psychiatrists (Patel *et al.* 2005). Nurses have also fallen into the trap that visiting patients to give them their depot constitutes the totality of the intervention. We see this with depot clinics or 'the two-weekly depot visit'. Nurses go and see patients because the depot falls on that day. This may be a legitimate use of the nurses' time, although this way of thinking fuels the suspicion that depot medication contributes towards 'old fashioned' methods of delivering psychiatric treatment.

Nurses are in a unique position to understand the method and science behind the giving of depot medication (Hamblet 2000). Nurses are particularly skilled in finding out the best ways to persuade patients to take their medication and often it is the nuances of the interaction that give insight into how patients are responding to their treatment. We know that giving medication does not substitute for the range of psychological treatments that go alongside the role of medication.

The overriding message is that patients should be informed of the various side effects of depot and oral medication and they should be offered a choice. One way to base this choice is to examine how drugs work in the body by looking at the receptor profiles for each individual drug. Examining how the drug works will give an indication on potential side effects. A number of case studies have chronicled the process to engage in a 'choice' agenda with mental health patients (Jones & Jones 2008a,b).

However, nurses themselves do not agree that patients should 'have the final say' in treatment (Harris *et al.* 2007). To add to this, if nurses believe medication (in this case, clozapine) is a viable and effective treatment option, compliance by patients with their medication increases (Angermeyer *et al.* 1999). To conclude, nurse prescribers need to hold at bay their own personal views on medication and to embrace a collaborative model in an effort to further the choice agenda.

Self-administration of medication

The administration of medication by patients themselves in hospital settings has been an area of nursing development for some time. Helping patients to self-administer their own medication helps to establish a framework to identify patients who may have problems managing or adhering to their own medication regime, and also helps to maintain and develop patient independence (Grantham *et al.* 2006). Patient self-administration is a key consideration for a nurse prescriber. In hospital settings, a role for nursing staff would be to assess whether patients are able to self-administer their own medication and to see how much support patients would require. Some organisations have developed levels of self-administration where medicines are locked in a cabinet or ward trolley and the key is kept by the nursing staff. At administration time the nurse instructs the patient how much of each drug to self-administer and then supervises the process, that is the nurse watches the patient taking the medication. It seems odd to think why self-administration has taken so long to be accepted as legitimate business in psychiatry given that it is patients themselves who have to take the medication when they go home.

Monitoring the side effects of medication

Many people fail to take their medication because of side effects caused by the treatment. This is a subject nurse prescribers must not avoid. The side effects that occur with psychotropic drugs and drugs for substance misuse are likely to impact on the physical and mental health of patients. Methadone, for example, is a drug that when given in large quantities causes respiratory depression. Haloperidol has a narrow index before causing movement disorder. The important point for nurses is to be able to identify and diagnose the adverse drug reaction so that remedial action can be considered and implemented (Bennett *et al.* 2005).

In order to do this, nurses need to be able to use a range of scales and profiles. You need to be selective in the type of rating scale and to be clear on why you wish to use it and how often. The benefit of a global scale is that it will broadly cover the metabolic and neurological adverse effects.

Some rating scales need prior training and require interpretation of information contained in medical notes, and are time-consuming (Lingjaerde *et al.* 1987). A helpful scale designed to be used by nurses is the West Wales Adverse Drug Reaction Profile, which includes the taking of vital signs, metabolic data, as well as observations and questions across neurological domains (Jordan *et al.* 2004). Other scales can be self-administered by the patient, for example the Liverpool University Neuroleptic Side Effect Rating Scale (LUNSERS) (Day *et al.* 1995b).

Useful time can be invested in finding out patients' concerns about taking medication and what control they think they have over the side effects. Nurses

> **Case Study**
>
> Jane is an independent nurse prescriber who decides to restart risperidone for a patient diagnosed with schizophrenia, who has just been admitted into hospital. Jane decides to carry out a baseline review of the patient's abnormal movements. Jane already notices that the patient has a fine tremor occurring in both hands when she first greets the patient.
>
> There are a number of scales to review abnormal movements, including the Barnes Akathisia Scale (Barnes 1989) and the Simpson–Angus Scale (Simpson & Angus 1970). Jane decides to use the Simpson–Angus Scale because it is designed specifically to detect extrapyramidal side effects. The scale has 10 questions and takes approximately 10 min to complete. Risperidone is known to cause muscular discomfort, and the patient has suffered from it when he was prescribed a higher dose of the drug to control his breakthrough symptoms.
>
> Jane also decides to give the patient a copy of the LUNSERS (Day *et al.* 1995b). This scale is self-administered and covers a wide array of possible symptoms along with some red herring items such as 'itchy skin'. The scale is useful in that it helps patients to identify with their own treatment plan and obtain a sense of control over their medication.

need to be mindful that patients may not have been asked before what they think about side effects and may find it difficult to talk about them. They may have received unsympathetic responses in the past. Herein lies the potential for nurses to form engagement strategies that foster control over medication.

It is likely that some nurse prescribers know their patients very well. This may lead some nurses to fail to spot certain side effects as they begin to develop. Other side effects of a greater magnitude may be missed because they have become 'normal' within the person's presentation. The side effects therefore get missed or minimised. To overcome this bias, patients should be examined by another nurse or psychiatrist with the expectation that side effects would be reviewed.

Advance directives

Not all people who suffer from mental health problems will elect to take medication when they are acutely disturbed. However, nurse prescribers must work for the development of individualised medication care plans – when people are well and fall ill. A weighing up of the pros and cons of taking medication in difficult circumstances is a natural process that we would all undertake. Nurse prescribers may wish to discuss with patients the role of advanced treatment directives should they become ill again through not taking medication (Healthcare Commission 2006). Nurse prescribers can talk through a range of

---

Case Study

Jack is 30 and has been suffering from paranoid schizophrenia for the last 11 years. Jack has frequent relapses because he defaults on taking medication. He has suffered from such severe relapses that he ends up being nursed in a psychiatric intensive care unit. He often receives acuphase [licensed to treat acute behavioural disturbance (BNF 2008)] and then quickly recovers so that he can be transferred back to an open ward. Jack was once denied this treatment and was treated with oral haloperidol [licensed for the treatment of psychomotor agitation (BNF 2008)] and his recovery period was prolonged. An advanced treatment directive was agreed with Jack by his nurse prescriber that if he became unwell he was to be prescribed acuphase.

---

treatments and, importantly, what treatment type to avoid if they presented in an emergency situation. Even when the crisis is abated, patients may still be unwell to make informed decisions about their treatment. An advanced treatment directive however could spell out the preferred treatment.

Conclusion

The harsh reality for psychiatric services is that up to 50% of patients who are prescribed psychotropic medication do not take it (Nose *et al.* 2003). Reasons are multifaceted and an approach is required that should be multimodal and flexible. The ability to impart choice in medicines management is a key indicator and a skill required for effective nurse prescribing. There are still many examples of a custodial approach taken by many mental health professionals, and this systemic approach is likely to crush any attempts by nurse prescribers to foster choice in the relationship. Helping patients to understand why they need to take medication may take longer during the consultation, although the benefits of this for the patient may appear further down the care pathway. There may be clinical situations were patients do need a behavioural approach, but this should not be the norm.

Encouraging patients to take their medication is complex and needs to be understood from the individual's perspective. The problems that otherwise result may have negative impacts on the patient's health and their wider social network and social environment. This is why nurse prescribers need to take on multiple interventions to help understand why patients wish to take medication or why not and how the nurse prescriber can best ensure that the prescribing relationship is collaborative and therapeutic.

Chapter 9
Nurse prescribers working as part of a team

Introduction

The reality of psychiatric care today is that nurse prescribers work as part of a team across the whole spectrum of mental health services. Professional groups working together produce benefits such as sharing of views and shaping of the clinical intervention from different disciplines in their endeavour to work with the complexity of mental health. On the opposite side, if teams become dysfunctional, clinicians can also raise and sustain conflict that prevent new roles new ways of delivering treatment from entering mainstream practice.

Nurse prescribing by its very nature will serve to confront long-held views on what certain professions do and should do in the future. In order to understand the dynamics of teamwork, some of factors that impede, sustain, nurture and add quality to the hotbed of what makes up teamwork will be discussed. Some, if not all, of these factors will impact on how nurse prescribing will be viewed by all mental health professionals.

The focus of this chapter will be to help nurse prescribers understand some of the small politics going on within teams. To this end, the chapter will not dwell on the larger political overtones that have driven or impeded the growth of nurse prescribing, albeit to acknowledge that nurse prescribing is a political tool progressed by a number of lobby groups (Jones 2004). Nurse prescribing raises issues about how care delivery is organised, the impact on present and future multidisciplinary team working and the roles of healthcare staff in the future. A potential paradox of nurse prescribing is that policy documents state that co-ordination between healthcare professions would improve (DoH 2003). What may be found is that nurse prescribing erodes professional boundaries or shifts the professional domain in how nurses and doctors work in the future. Nurses may try to assert themselves and negotiate an alternative position in the team in terms of their status and authority.

What is all the fuss about?

The nurse-prescribing journey is said to bring about better use of nurses' skills and knowledge within the team. However, doctors have been at times scathing about the approach. The British Medical Association expressed concerns about the safety of allowing nurses to prescribe medication (Avery & Pringle 2005). Other doctors have called the extension of prescriptive authority as 'embarking on a dangerous uncontrolled experiment' and 'reckless' (Horton 2002, page

1875). The USA has witnessed medical acceptance of nurse prescribing as long as some form of supervision takes place. This is also what has happened in the UK with supplementary prescribing. Doctors agree on the clinical management plan before medication can be prescribed and this acts as a vehicle to supervise and control nurse prescribers.

Some nurse academics have also been equally appalled by mental health nurses taking on prescriptive authority. There is a viewpoint that mental health nurses should reject the traditional and dominant medical model (Laungani 2002) that has been part of mental health services in general (Dawson 1997). Nurses equally worry that the core values of nursing or the practice of nursing will be distorted and eventually abandoned if they continue down the road becoming an extended arm of medicine. The question is whether these headline views will subside with time when wider teams begin to experience the benefits of nurse prescribing and clinicians see that nurses do not harm their patients. Evidence from the USA seems to indicate this (Kaas *et al.* 1998). However, there is a seismic shift occurring in what teams expect nurses to do. Nurse prescribing will challenge the philosophical basis of nursing being a care-focused activity.

Maybe the fuss has something to do with how the medical profession is presently defining itself or not. It may be that doctors are now finding it difficult to define what they do and experience a sense of dissatisfaction and a feeling of being under siege by other encroaching professional groups. The question is whether we still need doctors at all. The answer is obviously in the affirmative because they offer expertise above and beyond the advanced training undergone by nurses. However, this does not stop doctors from being suspicious about other professions encroaching on their role. The erosion of boundaries across all professional groups is happening constantly. However, professional erosion and threat also give the opportunity to state explicitly what you want nurses and doctors to do. The appropriate question here is: what is it that only a nurse or a doctor can do?

A forerunner to the question of what doctors did was their unqualified control over diagnosis and treatment. Nurse prescribing, which requires the ability to make a diagnosis and formulate a treatment plan, requires the same skills once held by doctors. That is why nurse prescribing has been seen as a threat to the authority and sense of purpose of being a doctor.

So who does the prescribing now?

One has to start off with who usually carries out prescribing responsibilities in teams. For some teams that have a close attachment, or part of primary care, the general practitioner may be the prescriber. For teams in hospital or secondary care, the prescriber is likely to be the psychiatrist. However, there is more to the prescribing decision than writing the prescription. Prescribing is more likely to be, or should be, a team effort if different professions and agencies are involved in the patient care. Psychiatrists are likely to listen and take on board issues raised by individual team members before taking their prescribing decision. General practitioners are most often guided by the suggestions made to them by mental health nurses and psychiatrists.

When mental health nurses are asked, they are able to identify the administration of medication and monitoring of side effects as one of their main roles (O'Brien & Cole 2004). Nurses have been administering medication because it was first used to treat people with mental illness. They have also advised medical staff on what to prescribe. At times, and understandably not documented, nurses have also given more or less medication than is charted, depending on the symptoms displayed by patients. There are also instances where nurses have given or told patients to take medication that has not been prescribed by a doctor. This may be the nurse telling the patient to take a higher or lower dose of the prescribed drug. This is de facto prescribing, but the extent of this practice would be difficult to uncover, given that it is unlawful. An argument can be made that the legislation behind nurse prescribing simply formalises what nurses have been doing for years.

Doctors are complicit in nurses prescribing medication in a de facto manner. Again it would be difficult to uncover the extent of this practice. A usual scenario would be for the nurse to make the medication adjustment and then inform the doctor. The doctor then authorises the medication change and so backdates the prescription to fit the date. The interesting question that emerges from the very essence of teamwork is why some nurses work in this way and not others. It strikes at the heart of the nurse–doctor relationship. On the one hand, the doctor trusts the nurse to make the correct clinical judgement because inevitably, the doctor would be covering for the nurse if problems emerged in the decision. On the other, the relationship supports a level of subservience between nurses and doctors that has been described for decades. In order for the nurse to act in this way, there must have been some implicit confidence expressed by the doctor for the nurse to act in this way. The doctor must have granted the nurse permission to work in this way. Such a discourse illustrates the complexity of teams that cannot be so easily separated out in what nurses, doctors and other professions do in their everyday life.

When nurses prescribe medication in a de facto manner, they must do it because of the perceived efficiency in getting medicines quicker to the patient. This may be correct for the majority of decisions. However, you have to question whether the ease of prescribing may always bring about better medicines management.

Another form of proxy prescribing is the use of pro re nata (as required) (PRN) medication in hospital settings. The frequency of prescribing PRN medication in hospital settings is large with very little guidance on how it should be policed (Baker *et al.* 2007). Without the use of PRN medication, junior doctors would be requested to prescribe medication frequently. When patients are prescribed PRN medication, nurses take the decision to give medication to them. There is a question about whether PRN medication is helpful to patients in all situations, but it is still used and is a way of prescribing by proxy.

A common and accepted norm of practice is where senior nursing staff working out of hours sees patients for assessment and then advises a junior doctor to prescribe medication. Most often, the nursing staff will have arrived at a safe and competent assessment and treatment plan. They may not have wider medical knowledge on systems, how diseases and treatments coexist or treatment. The junior doctor, on the other hand, is more likely to have awareness but not the depth of knowledge on diseases. If they are at Foundation doctor stage 1 or 2, they are extremely unlikely to have any experience in psychiatry or the effects of psychiatric drugs. Therefore, we have a ludicrous situation where senior nursing staff is taking prescribing decisions and then telling junior doctors to write the prescriptions. What has just been described is not without its benefits. For example, junior doctors are learning about the types of drugs to be given to patients most often in acute or emergency situations. Nursing staff can use this way of working as a platform to extend their practice or take on extended roles. However, let us not pretend that modern services should be planned and delivered on this basis and pretent that patients are well served by it.

Nurse prescribing is a new form of prescriptive authority that can potentially offer greater choice and access for patients. Its promise is to better maximise the skills of the team. For those nurses who go on to prescribe medication, there may be professional competition and tensions. Nurses are generally positive about nurse prescribing. However, doctors are not so positive. They express concerns about erosion of their professional roles and their position within the team. Doctors are particularly concerned about the safety of nurse and pharmacist prescribing in relation to their diagnostic skills (Hobson & Sewell 2006).

Nature of teams

Teams are commonly composed of nurses, social workers, occupational therapists and psychiatrists. These statutory professions sit alongside nonprofessional services and support agencies. All will have their own ways to determine assessment and will view patients differently (Jones 2006b). Historical, philosophical and theoretical underpinnings serve to draw distinctions among the members of the team. Hence the value of teams is their different viewpoints and interventions that can be offered (Onyett 2002). Nursing as a profession is central to the ethos of teams and is largely the dominant profession in terms of numbers within them. However, psychiatrists are often seen as the leaders of the teams in terms of their expertise in knowledge and patient management.

Nurses not only have always worked as part of a team in hospital settings but also as part of a wide range of community settings. The very nature of teams is to set in place structures and processes to help control and deliver care. All teams have their own ways to control referrals and manage work allocation, which has led to the concept of 'gate-keeping'. Gate-keeping brings into focus just exactly what you want professions to do with the referrals and to manage them through the system. When resources are stretched, the often 'sacred cows' of what professions do are broken down and you find community nurses leading outpatient reviews. Other examples are nurse consultants taking clinical responsibility for some aspects of inpatient care and nurse practitioners managing the often-complex array of factors when adults and older people present with a psychiatric emergency at the accident and emergency department in general hospitals. Examples like these scatter the seeds of opportunity. Some grow and develop into sustainable pathways of care, while others wither and are taken over by new ideas. In other words, different professional groups working together ultimately bring about a tension to handle aspects of care differently. The eclectic nature of nursing has used this hotbed as a springboard to advance all kinds of nurse-led interventions and services.

Essentially, teams are not homogenous collectives of people. Relations between and with team members have been dissected and studied for decades. In essence, disciplines tend to work according to set professional boundaries, and this tends to limit their awareness and appreciation of what other professional groups do within the patient care episode. The obvious example is diagnosis and treatment. Once the domain of medical staff, this is now being challenged with emerging evidence that nurses and lay people can be trained to diagnose and treat a range of conditions (Brugha *et al.* 1999a,b).

We frequently find nurses choosing to disinvest themselves of a view on patient care. In response, psychiatrists take on their role as responsible and experienced clinicians. Samson (1995) found that psychiatrists believed themselves to be superior to their team colleagues. Lazaro *et al.* (2001) concluded that psychiatrists perceived themselves as having a clinical responsibility for patients while other team members understood this responsibility to be shared (in the context of a crisis team). The underbelly of this point is who is responsible for the aspects of patient care and the ability of nurses and doctors to position themselves along the continuum of being responsible or not, as the case may be.

All teams show nurses and psychiatrists showing attributes described above, as there is always the potential for professional groups to revert to a comfort zone and be defensive if challenged. Nurse-led care and nurse prescribing will further challenge roles as new services are organised. The following case scenario illustrates how role change can lead to role conflict within the same profession.

Case Study

Jim was admitted to hospital with schizophrenia. The inpatient nursing team did not think his relapse was so severe that he needed inpatient treatment. The independent nurse prescriber who had been part of the admission process disagreed and felt inpatient care was appropriate and that a rechallenge of clozapine [licensed for the treatment of schizophrenia (BNF 2008)] was required. The independent prescriber not only had a responsibility to treat the patient safely but also had to counter the views of nursing staff that the patient should be discharged.

Traditionally, the psychiatrist would have been fending off the inpatient nursing staff, but with the change in role, it became more appropriately the role of the independent nurse prescriber. This adds in a new skill set for the nurse prescriber in being able to negotiate with nurses as part of a team effort when differences in opinion do not demarcate along traditional professional lines.

The practice of teamwork is possibly made difficult because of the contrasting positions that disciplines hold on a range of issues. For example, Patterson & Hayes (1977) found that disciplines adopted a particular occupational language developed during a period of professional training (Melia 1987). Teamwork could be affected when disciplines choose to align themselves to particular ways of discussing care or focusing on issues that are perceived relevant to them (Hamilton *et al.* 2004). Particular views such as the medical model may dominate the process and outcome of teamwork (Opie 1997). It is also important to unpack the different perspectives that clin-icians hold on the treatment of mental illness. Traditionally, psychiatric nurses have been negative towards the concepts associated with the medical model (Laungani 2002) and have abandoned the physical aspects of caring for people with mental illness. This has led some nurse academics to criticise the lack of 'biology' taught at the preregistration nursing level (Gournay 1995) and the chief nursing officer (DoH 2006c) to re-emphasise the importance of physical health monitoring and treatment. The irony of this historical failing is that the nursing profession is on the verge of taking on care roles that are closely aligned to medicine that the difference in role will merge even closer.

Is teamwork effective?

Teams have been part of mental health services for decades. In fact, we have witnessed an explosion of teams with the obsession of the NHS to splinter professional groups and large teams and what they do. All guidance, stretching back just under a decade, stress the value of multidisciplinary teams (DoH 1999c, 2008c). When groups of clinicians deliver care, outcomes improve for the patient (Zwarenstein & Reeves 2006). Particularly to medication, prescribing decisions actually improve when pharmacists work as part of the team as opposed to being a detached appendage working outside the team (Schmidt *et al.* 1998). Teams, as opposed to clinicians working in isolation, also have an effect on patient engagement (Burns & Lloyd 2004) and prevention of untoward incidents. So in this regard, teamwork can be effective as long as the different professional groups are clear about what they are doing for the patient (Barker & Walker 2000).

However, there are many examples where teams, if left unchecked, become unclear on what they have been set up to do. An example is the community mental health team, the demise of which has led to crisis resolution home treatment teams to manage the crisis element of health care and the assertive community treatment teams to manage the difficult-to-engage portion. The fact that such teams have atomised health care and left patients and staff bemused about who does what is a different matter.

Another example is modern hospital care and the control of clinical risks. Community mental health teams and specialist community teams place people in or out of hospital and the system is unable to regulate itself so that patients are able to stay for the right amount of time (Bowles & Jones 2005). It is professions themselves that control the system. Wrapped up in all of this is professional control over who decides care and treatment (Jones 2006b). This indeed is the real battleground, and for some clinicians, nurse prescribing will be like a touch flame to spilt paraffin.

Professional control

There is a whole sociological argument about how dominant professions control weaker professional groups in health care (Turner 1987). This manifests as to who controls the patient or what are the elements of health care to be treated and by whom (Cott 1998; Davies 2000; Coffey & Jenkins 2002). To coin a phrase from Foucault (1974), 'clinical gaze' is where health professions construct and determine what areas of health care they will deliver and engage in ways to limit that of other professions.

Psychiatrists themselves have reflected on their own shortcomings in being seen as the agents of control. Moncrieff (1997) looked at how organised psychiatry was resurgent in the range of drugs that were said to work for depression and schizophrenia. Psychiatrists have been employed and are complicit in controlling the deviants of society.

Psychiatrists have not just wanted to control patients. Poole & Bhugra (2008) have defended psychiatrists as being under siege by opportunistic professionals such as nurses who wish to wrestle control away for responsibilities such as prescribing. Rightfully so, there main concern is about patient safety. There are also similar arguments that medicine has been robbed of its rightful place in being the guarantors of medical examination and diagnosis (Craddock *et al.* 2008). One can conclude that psychiatry is in a professional turmoil as it adapts to the changing needs of patients.

It is not the purpose of this book to dwell on the negative impact on the excessive overtones of this position but to acknowledge its presence. However, it is important to cover ways in which members of the healthcare team perceive nurse prescribers in both a negative and positive light because this has implications for nurses who wish to prescribe medication.

One must accept that not all clinicians are in favour of nurse prescribing for a number of reasons. There is a line of argument that psychiatrists have managed health care since the days of asylum. Historically, medical superintendents had authority to employ and dismiss nursing staff or attendants, as they were so called. Although ministerial papers and the Mental Health Act changed the responsibility and accountability framework, nurses still perceive the authority of medical staff. In many respects, this is a reflection of the way society at large views the medical profession. With perceived authority comes control. Such control may act as a driver for nurses to prescribe medication and can be used to obtain positive effects. For example, nurses may be discouraged from prescribing by line managerial reluctance but are supported by influential med-ical staff. However, the double edge may come into play where medical staff are opposed to nurse prescribing and prevent its adoption.

Some clinicians feel that their professional training is more in depth and they had to study for a long time to achieve the success and control that their post gives them. Professional knowledge and control over this knowledge by one professional group over another may inhibit the growth of nurse prescribing. An obvious example is between medical and nursing staff. Entry qualifications for initial study and continuing study are vastly different. Claims of clinical knowledge and experience being more superior to others are played out in teams both directly and indirectly.

In teams where nurses prescribe medication in a de facto fashion, psych-iatrists permit them to work in this way. They allow nurses to exercise their judgement, and there is a knowing acceptance that if untoward errors occur, a degree of collusion will be entered into. At the heart of this dynamic is power and control.

One can argue that control by the medical profession over nurse prescribing has been supported through the present policy on supplementary prescribing. Psychiatrists decide what can be prescribed and to whom. Indeed, the National Prescribing Centre (2005a) advocated that psychiatrists and nurses start off with limited clinical management plans and then progress on to more liberated medication plans. In other words, as competency is developed and displayed to psychiatrists, the shoestrings of what the nurse prescriber can prescribe would become looser but never cut. This play on words revolves around control.

Professional fragmentation

Teamwork also gives rise to clinicians taking on practices once previously completed by other discipline groups. This arises through the organisation using the most appropriate skill set to achieve the desired outcome and a need for generic working. The concept of shared skills has been put forward with *The Capable Practitioner* (Sainsbury Centre for Mental Health 2001). Distributed responsibility and shared decision making have been advanced through new ways of working (DoH 2005b). We have also seen the introduction and extension of the European Working Time Directive and the revolution this has had on what junior doctors do now and will do in the future. As professions fragment and adapt, resistance is encountered that can spill out in thwarting developments such as nurse prescribing. Many policy documents outline how nurses can add a nursing dimension to a whole range of tasks previously carried out by medical staff, particularly for chronic diseases (DoH 2005a).

Teamwork also raises particular challenges in terms of who does w[...]
patients. Traditionally, psychiatrists decided the treatment plan and [...]
administered it. Some nursing staff were happy for this role to be enacted[...]
varying degrees. It also enabled some nurses and doctors to take positions i[...]
the team, which allowed them to express their opinion or allowed particular
clinicians to advocate taking or not taking medication. With nurse prescribing,
nurses may well be the clinicians who are advocating the need for treatment and
expecting their colleagues to administer it.

Some would argue that medicine has a strong sense of identity about what
it does and the value placed on what it does by society. An argument could be
made that the public values the doctor–patient relationship in the sense that
doctors are viewed as competent to find out what is wrong with them and then
give the treatment. This social construct may not be there for nursing as yet
and one must question whether it will ever be. The public may not see a nurse
prescriber as being as competent as a medical prescriber. Essentially, the public
sees nursing as being about caring and the nursing profession sustains this viewpoint. Nurse prescribing is not constructed to fit within this paradigm, so this
may fuel professional disputes and rivalry between doctors and nurses.

Professional disputes and rivalry

Inevitably, developments such as nurse prescribing and autonomous practice
will give rise to boundary disputes where professions become defensive about
certain parts of their care. Beattie (1995) suggested that clinicians developed a
'tribalistic' culture, which preserves professional power and uniqueness of occupational identity. However, this position is constantly under threat with challenges currently being worked through for psychiatrists in just exactly what
aspect of care different professions should be managing. New ways of working for psychiatrists (DoH 2005b) and mental health nurses (DoH 2006c) are
driving at full speed ahead through the vehicle of what was the old-fashioned
concept of traditional roles. The important aspect of nursing is that they are
able to articulate their viewpoint. It is a concern that nurses do not feel assertive
enough to do so (DoH 2006c) and this must be considered when they start to
take on prescribing responsibilities in the future.

It may well be found that nurse prescribing helps clinicians to work in partnership between medical and nursing colleagues. Nurse prescribing may bring about
efficiencies so that psychiatrists do not need to spend much time examining people when this work could be performed for them by nurse prescribers. Some could
argue that when nurses carry out this way, it is a return to the medical model. One
could take the opposite view that nurses are taking patients out of the medical
model and providing them with an experience closer to their social context.

Nurse prescribers will also be faced with situations when their responsibility for patient care does not lead to an outcome as expected by the team.
When prescribing decisions 'go wrong', nurses will face chinks in the armour

...und knowledge about diseases, mental state and psychophar-
...es may have to face the claim that their knowledge base did not
...ke on aspects of care and treatment. Situations like these will
...r because psychiatry is not an exact science. In many situa-
...right answer and prescribing clinicians do not know a priori
...work. The problem for nurse prescribers is that they will be
... defending a prescribing decision within this morass of uncertainty.

One of the stated advantages of nurse prescribing is that it helps teams to deliver better care because prescribers are more accessible to patients (DoH 2006c). Now better care could be care that is delivered by the right person at the right time. However, the issue here is that the team itself will have different views on what this statement actually means. Team members may actually feel uncomfortable as potentially being usurped by a nurse prescriber. This feeling may actually cut across all members of the multidisciplinary team. Team members may feel as though their area of practice or their field of specialty is being threatened by the development of nurse prescribing. This is precisely why nurses need to understand the culture of psychiatric teams so that they can begin to navigate how nurse prescribing can work effectively.

Clinicians may perceive that they are in competition with nurse prescribers or nurse prescribers may think they are in competition with junior doctors or even consultants. Nurses may try and pit their social knowledge of patients (deemed as more in depth than the consultant) against the broader medical knowledge held by psychiatrists. Such tensions may well lead to conflict and inevitably poor patient care.

There is a strong body of opinion that questions why nurses should take on prescriptive authority. Various reasons can be spelt out to support this conclusion and can be played out in the way teams work. For example, a nurse prescriber may be working with a patient deciding treatment and overseeing patient care. Another nurse in the team who has negative views on nurse prescribing may then turn to the consultant psychiatrist for an opinion on the way forward. This way of working and thinking ultimately undermines the prescriptive autonomy of the nurse prescriber. Now it is up to the psychiatrist to resist this dialogue and to refer the nurse to the nurse prescriber, but it may not be so easy to identify, given the various ways by which clinical information or requests for advice can be sought.

Views on mental illness and disability: Models, muddles and medicine

Teams bring with them their own philosophical and theoretical views on health, disease, illness and treatment thereof (Tyrer & Steinberg 2005). This is commonly referred to as the model of care. In mental health, teams often throw around the concept of the disease or medical model, social model, psychodynamic model and cognitive behavioural model. We will focus on the medical and social models because these have direct relevance to nurse prescribing.

The medical model in its purest form suggests that a disease arises from a physiological cause. An established system of examination, symptom description, treatment and prognosis of disease is the bedrock of medicine (Tyrer & Steinberg 2005). The problem for nursing is that the medical model is caricatured as something that is bad and corrupt within teams. Some clinicians react against nurse prescribing because it is seen as supporting the medical model (Snowden 2007). Viewing patients' diseases or illnesses as having some pathological cause in isolation to their social and psychological state misrepresents the basis of psychiatric nursing and psychiatry in general. However, the negative associations attached to the medical model are played out in teams routinely.

The social model has gained huge attraction as a guiding framework in our management of mental illness. People from poorer households are more likely to suffer depression and anxiety. We also face an economic necessity to bring people back to work and to reduce the sickness benefit culture. It is correct to champion the social model to help people in society to better manage the problems they face and also for society to lessen the burden of them. However, we find some clinicians to extol this model as though it is at odds with anything else that is not social. Nurse prescribers may find themselves working alongside people who reject what they do because of the supposed conflicts with the social model. However, nurse prescribing is not antithesis to the social model, rather the contrary, if we just reflect again on the early studies on nurse prescribing (Luker *et al.* 1998). Patients like nurses to prescribe because they do it within a social context, with a social discourse that engages patients.

Nurse prescribing naturally brings the work of nurses into a closer alignment with the medical aspects of patients' presentation simply because medication is being proposed as a possible treatment. A charge that can be levelled at the nurse-prescribing agenda is that nurses will be taken into the medical model even further than before. One could argue that nurses need to have a much further in-depth knowledge of patients' physical health and how common diseases coexist with mental illness.

The medical model is associated with superiority of the doctor, the role of the doctor being the expert in diagnosis, treatment and the general direction of care (Lanceley *et al.* 2007). Doctors take the attitude of being superior in relation to nurses and patients. If nurse prescribing is associated with the medical model, then nurse prescribers may assume some of these attributes and replicate the negative associations. However, in defence of this assertion, studies investigating the social discourse of nurse prescribing suggest that patients prefer to talk to nurses about their medication needs, compared to doctors (Jones *et al.* 2007).

Nurse prescribers may also face criticism from nurses and other team members who profess models of care that support social or psychological explanations for symptoms and treatment. Nurse prescribers may end up having grandstanding conversations about the merits and demerits of models over others. With the medical model, nurse prescribers may try to minimise the negative associations of the medical model as though it is devoid of social and psychological aspects. Nurse prescribers may enter into this discourse unintentionally, but a tug-of-war may develop in trying to offer the best explanation for the illness and treatment. Nurse prescribers need to start off with a simple explanation of the medical model as being a bio-socio-psycho orientation that helps them in their work to diagnose and treat patients.

Nurse prescribers must also bear in mind that the true essence of teams is that their nature is made up of different personalities and ways of thinking about mental health. Clinicians will choose to adopt certain positions over others. It seems unlikely that a clinician who espouses the social model would enrol on the prescribing course for instance. It is important that nurse prescribers appreciate that no theoretical model explains in totality the treatment of mental illness and various disorders.

What impact will nurse prescribing have on other team members and the functioning of the team?

The relationships that nurse prescribers have within teams, the impact of team working and support from within the team will all have an impact on the successful take-up of this initiative. It has been established that it is best for nurses to take prescribing decisions as part of a team. However, will nurse prescribing make the patient experience any better? Will it be more efficient? Will the decisions be correct in terms of diagnosis and treatment formulation? In terms of patient satisfaction, patients like to see a nurse prescriber probably because of the amount of time and the type of discourse that they have with nurses. In terms of efficiency, there may be a variation compared to psychiatrists. Psychiatrists will have perfected the art of diagnostic interviewing, enabling them to carry out their examination to arrive at the correct formulation. It is not in the tradition for nurses to perform diagnostic interviews, essential for independent prescribing and helpful for supplementary prescribing. Therefore nurses may be slower to carry out their assessments. They may also not possess the same level of competence of doctors, so the diagnostic conclusions may be incorrect (notwithstanding the position that doctors also make diagnostic errors). Only time in training will enable nurses to carry out diagnostic interviews at the speed seen by the psychiatrist. However, one has to consider the patient who is exposed to this activity. One of the very strengths of nursing is that they can talk to patients that may lead to interventions being accepted in a more receptive manner.

We have many commentaries from medical staff that nurse prescribing is not safe and that a calamity will occur at some stage. Medical staff may well have fears about the safety of patients but a question that must be considered is whether they are also worried about the identity of the medical profession for themselves. As yet there has been little research in the UK that has documented the effect that nurse prescribing will have on what doctors do, what patients they will see or, if nurse prescribing actually improves, the quality of prescribing undertaken.

Pharmacists are permitted to prescribe but the adoption has been relatively modest, particularly in the primary care setting (Guillaume *et al.* 2008). Why is this? Is it the best use of pharmacists' resources to be seeing patients, carrying out case management functions that go hand in hand with prescribing? There is a national shortage of mental health pharmacists; should this valuable highly trained resource be spent on actual prescribing or should they support nurses who prescribe through supervision? However, if pharmacists do not prescribe, then the question that needs to be asked is how they can understand the practicalities of prescribing. A thread running through this chapter and pertinent to pharmacists will be the impact of a further prescriber on the wider team and how roles will change as a result (Tonna *et al.* 2007).

Strategies to overcome team tensions

Nurse prescribers, first and foremost, must locate their practice within a team ethos. Understanding the basis of teams, how they function and how nurse prescribing could potentially work is fundamental. This factor alone may be one of the reasons why nurse prescribing fails to take place.

Nurses need to resist being snared in competitive rivalry with competing professional groups. Such activity is unhelpful not only for nurse prescribing but also for patient care. Nurses who have started the journey towards nurse prescribing need to form collaborative relationships with senior prescribers and learn from them. This is why some countries such as Ireland and the USA have formalised collaborative practice agreements between nurses and medical staff members. They state exactly what nurse prescribers can do and what supervision is in place.

Experienced clinicians are aware that roles are changing not only for all professions but also within the nursing profession. A study conducted in the USA noted that registered nurses not only respected nurse prescribers but also wanted to receive respect back for the ordinary role they provided (Gooden & Jackson 2004). Those who adopt new roles should be mindful that not all members of the team are necessarily going to be in agreement. Nurses should be proud to have prescriptive authority and to show respect for the wider nursing roles required for patient care. If not, it will work against them in terms of winning over staff colleagues.

Teams will begin to understand and appreciate the value of nurse prescribers when the actual activity of nurse prescribing brings about added value to patient care. There are instances where nurse prescribing takes place just so that prescribing activity takes place. This is not necessarily over prescribing or prescribing out of context. This is why the activity of nurse prescribing must meet the needs of the service as opposed to nurses prescribing because of the attraction in itself. One may need to look at how nurse prescribing has been implemented to understand implementation deficit. One of the main reasons why implementation deficit occurs is that prescriptive authority has been added on to the nurses' role without any consideration to the strategic context of benefit realisation.

It is inevitable that nurse prescribers will come across patients whose care and treatment is not so easy to define. The nurse prescriber may have insufficient skills to extract the information in which to base their pharmacological treatment plan. In this case, the nurse prescriber is responsible for passing over the patient back to the psychiatrist without delay. Now some nurse prescribers may feel that they have undermined their own self-worth in doing this. Obviously, the principles of patient safety come before self-appeasement in their endeavours to prescribe. However, this type of experience adds a certain advantage. Firstly, it establishes the supremacy of teams being made up of different professions with different levels of skill and ability. Secondly, it reinforces the principle that patients are not homogenous groups of patients with the same levels of need. Patients can shift back and forth depending on who can meet their needs best. Thirdly, it supports the position long held by policy rhetoric that nurses can manage a tier of patients but that a more select group of patients are best served by doctors (as part of a team).

Using teams and team functioning to help improve medicines management

Nurses must take on board and understand why medication-related errors occur for themselves and others. Nurses have a responsibility to collaborate with others in the prevention, management and reduction of medicines-related incidents. This is best performed within a whole systems approach.

All nurse prescribers will be working in some way with psychiatrists or a general practitioner either within a supplementary or within an independent prescribing relationship. The benefits of close collaboration will help to ensure the nurse maintains competence to prescribe. Nurses and doctors working within a team approach will separate out possibly sterile clinical issues that may be discussed in supervision from the actual live cases being managed by the team.

Wider teams within health organisations will also have specific medicines management groups set up to monitor medicines incidents. It is essential that nurse prescribers are represented on this group to learn from wider organisational issues and how it relates back to their own prescribing practice. Specifically, nurse prescribers would add to the value of drug and therapeutic committees, given their experience of prescribing.

Some evidence has shown that nurse prescribers are more likely to prescribe when peer support emanates from the team (Otway 2002). Effective interpersonal relationships held and sustained by nurse prescribers are essential to elicit support from the team. Hay *et al.* (2004) found that unless the teams support nurse prescribing, implementation will be difficult to sustain. Working in isolation impacted negatively on the person's confidence to prescribe. Ways to support peer support may be to train other nurses in the team to prescribe and increase team understanding on the important role of the nurse prescriber as part of team delivery of care.

An exciting area of development and one that holds promise for nurse prescribing is the work carried out on whole systems training called 'creating capable teams' (DoH 2007b). This is where a whole team approach is taken to decide what the team does to meet patient need, what type of professions and what numbers are required to meet the needs of patients. If one accepts that teams could benefit from employing a nurse prescriber, it seems likely that new roles and a training plan would emerge to take forward nurse prescribing. However, unless one is working in a dynamic team, it is unlikely that the team members themselves would come up with deciding to use nurse prescribing. Nurse prescribing is more likely to come about through an explicit process to look at roles, function and care delivery.

Teams have intelligence about the workflow of patients, who is best to see patients and how skills of the team can meet the burden of work. Ramcharan *et al.* (2001) noted very early on for mental health nurse prescribing that the complexity of the case for nurse prescribers needs to be worked through. Part of this conclusion is for teams and team members to work through together in deciding the cases most appropriate to be seen by the nurse prescriber. Nurse prescribing is an interdisciplinary intervention dependent on the team for cases and input to how cases should be managed.

When nurses prescribe medication, they do so not as individuals but as part of a team. Nurses need to remember this 'team' ethos when they prescribe medication, simply because information not passed on about the prescribing decision is potentially dangerous.

Conclusion

Nurse prescribing should be viewed as part of a wider team enterprise. Nurse prescribing has not been introduced as a driver to displace multidisciplinary team working, rather the opposite. If nurses end up working in isolation from the team, this will be a dangerous precedent. Teamwork acts as a safeguard against maverick clinicians who wish to go out and prescribe without considering the wider views of the team. Teams also help to educate clinicians on the varied and wide experiences of clinical situations that occur and that would not be experienced by single clinicians working on their own.

Clinicians from all professional backgrounds will express their views on how and where nurses will prescribe medication. Each professional group has vested interests to preserve the interests of their own professional standing. Hence, there are various problems in teams and teamwork that is evident in our healthcare and social care systems. Professional control, rivalry and erosion models of care have been discussed within the context of a nurse prescriber. Nurse prescribers need to work with the tensions that exist within teams and to steadily overcome them by being interpersonally aware and judging how best prescriptive authority can meet the needs of patients.

Chapter 10
Ethical and legal issues in mental health nurse prescribing

Introduction

The ethics and legal issues with nurse prescribing are intertwined. Nurses will need to have knowledge on the relevant legislation, professional obligations and employment requirements for them to practice ethically and legally. Each stage of the prescribing process can be subject to ethical and legal challenges. Nurse prescribing will challenge the existing boundaries of what nurses do for patients. Undoubtedly, political influences have shaped health care where the reality is that nurses take on more and more of the roles once undertaken by medical staff. This is a logical next step for nursing practice, hence the importance of examining the ethical and legal frameworks in which nurses will base their practice.

Healthcare ethics emanates from moral philosophy and guides how people should behave and conduct themselves. It is important for mental health nurses to realise that the ethical beliefs and standards may be different to patients. Putting it simply, patients may well have different views from professionals on medication, hence the importance of patient choice. When nurses and patients have differences in their opinions, difficulties in concordance are likely to take place. Ethical issues for mental health nursing are about the duties and responsibilities of mental health nurses towards patients to ensure that they follow the right course of action. Although the right course of action may not be deemed illegal, nurse-prescribing decisions may well have a different ethical dimension.

Legal framework

The prescription of medication is subject to law for all health professions. Before the 1990s, only doctors and dentists could prescribe medication as defined by the Medicines Act (1968) and the Misuse of Drugs Act (1971). Since then legal changes to who can prescribe and what can be prescribed have been amended through various primary and secondary legislation changes.

Since 2007, the primary legislation allowing nurses to prescribe medication is the Health and Social Care Act 2001. Within this Act, Sections 63 and 42 cover the extension of prescribing responsibilities. These sections amended the

Medicines Act 1968. The Health and Social Care Act 2001 also enabled the passing of ministerial powers through an order to:

- designate additional categories of prescribers;
- set conditions upon the scope of prescribing.

Nursing staff are permitted to prescribe medication through a supplementary and independent prescribing framework. Nurse prescribing, along with certain functions within the Mental Health Act (DH 2007b), is one of two nursing actions defined by Law.

As nurse prescribing is a legally defined action, it opens the case to claims of negligence and liability. Each of these terms will be explored in this chapter to give meaning for mental health nurses.

Expanding practice

Nurses have been expanding their role since new technologies emerged. New roles such as of nurse consultants and new amendments to the Mental Health Act (DoH 2008b) will force through further changes to what nurses do now and would do in the future. Nurse prescribing is a new and evolving practice. It is about nurses expanding their role into what was the sole domain of medicine. However, what must come with it is an appreciation of legal liability and professional accountability, and this is something that nursing has struggled with for some time. If we look back on the nursing profession, it seems to want responsibility for patient care, but when the situation becomes 'tricky', it takes an about-turn and abdicates decision making to the doctor in charge. You will often hear statements such as 'that's the doctor's decision' or 'lets wait for the doctor' when making decisions about discharge from service or hospital.

When situations go wrong

In all clinical situations, there are no a priori set of rules that guarantee a positive end point in treatment. This rule is never more true for mental health. It is the consequences of untoward incidents that we will focus on here. When an intervention is delivered that results in an unexpected outcome and is deemed to be negative, then it is classed as untoward. Some untoward incidents are serious to merit reporting for investigation. An investigation should be carried out to determine the presence of systemic failure as opposed to personal failure. However, not all clinicians perceive this when they experience the untoward incident process. One must keep in perspective that incidents do occur through no fault of the clinician. Most often they are systemic problems that can be rectified. However, when situations do go wrong, the system itself is opened up to scrutiny.

Clinical situations can occur with serious consequences for the patient. In these situations, the patient or the family may seek legal redress and attempt to prove negligence. Before they can prove negligence, legal redress first needs to establish liability.

This is why it is important for nurse prescribers to be aware that civil and criminal laws will not only help protect them as nurse prescribers but they will also protect patients whom they serve. The best way to understand how the laws are used in the UK is to apply case law and the best way to understand case law is to apply it to nurse prescribing.

Liability

Nurse prescribers are very concerned about how liable they would be if an untoward incident were to occur with their prescribing practice. Vicarious liability is defined as when a nurse prescriber, who is the employee, prescribes as part of their duties in the course of their employment. Under these circumstances, the employer is vicariously liable for the actions, errors and omissions of the prescriber. There are many examples of extended practice where nurses first take on activities once carried out by medical staff and where those activities are not authorised by the organisation. A challenge may occur where the employer has allowed the employee to carry out a range of interventions that are wrong. Organisations have tried to manage the activities of clinical staff by writing policies that determine what interventions people can do for the management of certain conditions.

One must be clear that when a nurse prescriber delivers an intervention, they are professionally and ethically accountable for the practice. The nurse prescriber never stops being accountable for their intervention or the omission of an intervention. If a nurse is employed by an organisation and they are delivering the intervention as part of their employment, then the employer is liable for any act or omission that leads to damage. This is why it is important and probably explains the reason why nurse prescribing has had a fitful start in some organisations across the UK. The essential point is that the nurse prescriber does not deliver those interventions for which they have not been trained, or in which they are not deemed competent. A nurse prescriber will not be able to claim lack of knowledge or a low level of competence as a defence in terms of a breach of duty of care.

It is important for nurse prescribers to realise that NHS organisations cannot abdicate their responsibilities for vicarious liability. If organisations put in place a policy for nurses to prescribe medication as part of their role, then they accept liability for the actions of the nurse who performs the role. Liability cannot be split where one part of the role is covered whilst another part is not.

Medical indemnity has been in place for many years. Nurses who hold and use prescriptive authority should ensure that they have professional indemnity insurance. Such means can come from trade union membership or a professional organisation. It is important that nurse prescribers have professional indemnity to cover them against criminal charges and professional disciplinary matters. Nurse prescribers need to be aware that they will each be liable for damages caused through their actions. Nurse prescribers need to ensure that they understand what their employing organisations mean by vicarious liability and how far this would extend to cases where practice undertaken is sometimes unclear. For example, if a breach in the duty of care were proved, the employing organisation may seek legal redress from the employee.

Negligence

Since the 1990s the rise in clinical negligence claims is alarming. For 2006–2007, there were just under 5500 claims of clinical negligence against the NHS. Just over half a billion was spent on clinical negligence for 2006–2007. For 2008, total liabilities for NHS negligence is in the region of 9 billion pounds (NHS LA 2008). It is estimated that there are 500 reported incidents a month but only 1% of these are deemed to be serious. The challenge of nurse prescribing therefore is whether the nurse prescribing activity will actually increase these costs or reduce them.

In the overall context of clinical negligence, mental health is of low risk but not an unsubstantial financial challenge to any organisation should the risk result in a clinical negligence claim. This may help explain why organisations may be restrictive in what nurses can prescribe and where in order to lower the risk of untoward incidents.

Clinical negligence is an act or omission that causes a patient harm. The process of civil law is concerned with compensating patients who have suffered harm as a result of an intervention. In order for clinical negligence to be proved, the following four points need to be established.

(1) A legal duty of care has been compromised.
(2) The defendant was in breach of the duty of care and did not reach the standard of care required by law.
(3) Care did not follow a logical procedure.
(4) The breach of duty caused or contributed to the damage suffered.

When a nurse uses their prescriptive authority with a patient, they are entering into a contract with the patient that implies consent (when the patient has given it) and authority to act. The patient who receives prescriptive advice has the right to receive their care to a set standard. The nurse also has a duty of care to give that advice. When this fact has been established, a failing in this duty of care is presided over by considering two more issues.

The first fact is to establish a duty of care and whether that duty of care as delivered by a nurse prescriber was upheld to a standard of their peers otherwise known as the Bolam Test. If the actions of the nurse prescriber fall short of acceptable standards then the courts could decide the issue of damage or injury as a result of the incompetent actions. Herein lays the second test called the Bolitho Test, which is to determine whether the standard can be defended logically. This places a legal duty on the nurse prescriber to keep themselves up-to-date and consider the body of evidence that is judged to be the standard for safe health care.

In relation to the Bolitho Test, the problem for nurse prescribers is that treatments do not always work the same and there are different ways to arrive at the process of care. We also know that the evidence base supporting psychiatric treatment is, at best, conflicting. There are plenty of examples where interventions are delivered in psychiatry without any evidence. The point to be made is that nurses must be able to defend whatever course of action they take and a consideration documented of the comparative risks of delivering one intervention over another.

A pressing concern amongst nurse prescribers is that they work as part of a team and that their prescribing practice is indeed supported by the team. Supplementary prescribing and the clinical management plan even suggest and lend support to the concept that the nurse and the doctor are working as a team given that they are both agreed on the diagnosis and the treatment plan. However, the reality is that in law there is no such thing as team liability. Each nurse prescriber is professionally and personally accountable for their actions.

The question that needs to be considered is whether a failing in the duty of care had been committed. One way to understand duty of care is to look at the process of prescribing. Failings leading to a breach in the duty of care may occur in the following areas.

(1) Taking a proper history and mental state
(2) Formulating a correct diagnosis
(3) Performing a satisfactory physical examination in relation to the presentation
(4) Ordering of appropriate tests and onward referrals
(5) Devising the clinical management plan
(6) Processing of prescription
(7) Referral to specialist advice when necessary

Case Study

Fred has been referred to the accident and emergency department by a general practitioner because he was feeling low in mood. He was seen by Jacky who worked in the liaison clinic and is an independent nurse prescriber. A full assessment as possible was undertaken and the first issue to be noted was of a mood disorder characterised by poor sleep, irritability and poor concentration. Fred was insistent on leaving the department and protested that all he needed was to go home to sleep and take rest. Jacky's treatment plan included the prescribing of zopiclone [drug licensed for insomnia (BNF 2008)] at a single dose of 7.5 mg and then to follow him up in the liaison clinic.

The following day, Fred self presented at the psychiatric unit. He complained of hearing voices commanding him to set fire to himself. He also sets fire to a bin in the courtyard of the hospital, which causes damage to the exterior wall of the hospital and leads to the fire brigade being called to put out the fire. In the process, Fred suffers 40% burns and takes his case to a solicitor to seek negligence on the part of the nurse prescriber.

This scenario identifies a number of important points about nurse prescribing. The first is accountability for one's actions. Nurses need to clearly document the extent of their assessment, and why certain actions were complete and not others. From the example above, the nurse prescriber would need to demonstrate through their actions why the patient was not admitted into hospital or offered support through a home treatment team and why the patient was offered a course of zopiclone.

Ethical theory

Ethical theory will help the nurse prescriber to think critically about the prescribing encounter. Two ethical theories of relevance for nurse prescribers are deontology and utilitarianism. The practice of ethics is supported by a number of ethical principles such as respect for autonomy for the patient or staff member.

Deontology

The main proponent of this approach was a German philosopher called Immanuel Kant. Kant's approach to deontology was based on human reason and strongly influenced by religious beliefs. A deontological approach is where ethical dilemmas are considered by adopting a duty-based approach in terms of how it affects not only the duty to the nurse prescriber but also the obligations to the patient, and to do this irrespective of the consequences of those actions. The merits of deontology are that all nurse prescribers would work to a high standard: where patients and staff would be comfortable knowing that they would receive their treatment according to set standards regardless of the consequences. The disadvantage of this approach is that obviously deontology disregards the consequences of the actions of the nurse prescriber.

Utilitarianism

Utilitarianism was put forward in the 19th century by the English philosophers Jeremy Bentham and John Stuart Mill. A utilitarian approach is where the nurse prescribers consider the consequences of their nurse prescribing decisions and take into consideration a course of action that would lead to the greatest good. A utilitarian approach leads to actions that result in the greatest good for the greatest number.

A scenario that a mental health nurse can best consider to delineate these two ethical principles is when one considers the cost of antipsychotic medication. It is known that any of the atypical drugs are considerably expensive compared to haloperidol, which is extremely cheap for the treatment of psychosis. With limited drug budgets, a nurse prescriber adopting a deontological approach may prescribe aripiprazole [drug licensed to treat bipolar disorder (BNF 2008)]

because it is an atypical drug, it has a kinder side-effect profile and it is me
the needs of the patient. A utilitarian approach is where nurse prescribers would
prescribe haloperidol because it is just as efficacious as other atypical drugs, it
is considerably cheaper and although it causes side effects, more patients can be
treated and resources can be spent on other forms of health care. This is the
simplest scenario to distinguish these two ethical principles, and it is the task of
the nurse prescriber to consider their conscience and the effect of the prescribing
decision on autonomy, beneficence and choice.

Autonomy

Clinical situations may occur where a patients' autonomy may be compromised
if they are not given the correct information about proposed treatment to enable
them to make an informed choice. For example, the product specification sheets on
medication leaflets goes through a whole range of possible side effects of medication, although in clinical use the nurse prescriber is unlikely to go through all those
potential problems. Patients' autonomy in this situation would be compromised.
This is why the nurse-prescribing initiative has been so successful. In the early nurse
prescribing research, patients complimented the social style of nurse prescribing
and the ability to understand information regarding the medicinal products (Luker
et al. 1998). If this can be contrasted with the medical consultation where patients
are given on average 7 min with their general practitioner, it seems improbable
that the correct information regarding diagnosis, treatment, side effects and likely
effects of medication can be adequately communicated to serve autonomy.

Autonomy can also be applied to nursing staff. There may be a conflict for
nurse prescribers in how other people see their role. For example, nurses and
doctors may hold the view that only medical staff are trained to diagnose and
prescribe medication and that nurses should refrain from such activity. Such
resistance may hamper the ability of nurses to exercise the full autonomous
practice of their new skill. There may well be some nurses and doctors who feel
that the amount of time and resources it takes for patients to receive medication
from a nurse prescriber is disproportionate to the gain achieved. In other words,
the time could be better spent in other areas of nursing practice.

With informed consent, it is assumed that patients are able to understand the
issues about medication and to exercise a will of judgement on their options.
Nurse prescribers must outline the choices regarding treatment and give sufficient information regarding side effects and the likely effects of nontreatment.
Patients often come to the clinical encounter with some background knowledge
of medication, either through experiencing it themselves or what they have read.
It would not be uncommon for someone to experience a relapse of their psychosis and to request more medication, or to request a choice or a change in their
medication and to give reasons why. Nurse prescribers will also have to contend
with situations where patients exert their choice not to take medication even
though, on balance, patients may well relapse.

Accountability and freedom to act

If one looks at accountability from an historical perspective, the act of nursing was seen as an extension of the medical arm of practice. Hence, accountability is a dynamic process that changes over time as practice develops. The nursing profession has recently updated its accountability framework in relation to medication management and nurse prescribing (Nursing & Midwifery Council 2006).

Accountability here means acquiring knowledge and skills to perform the nurse prescribing role as defined by being a supplementary or independent prescriber. The nurse is then held accountable for decisions and actions taken as a result of this particular set of interventions. The following case scenario helps to illuminate this point.

Case Study

Andy has set up a clinic in the general practitioner surgery where he takes referrals and carries out assessment and prescribing for patients with mild to moderate mental health conditions such as depression and anxiety. Andy has set up a system where the general practitioner not only first sees the patient and then triggers off a referral but also fills up a clinical management plan agreement form. Andy is then able to prescribe medication.

The patient has been seen by the general practitioner and a moderate depression is diagnosed, and has been referred to Andy's clinic for treatment and review. Andy agrees with the diagnosis of depression, follows the agreed treatment plans and signs off the management plan with the patient. Andy prescribes escitalopram [drug licensed for depression (BNF 2008)]. The patient then develops symptoms of sweating and agitation, which worsens the depression. The patient then attempts to commit suicide and is taken to accident and emergency department after 4 days of treatment.

This dilemma raises a number of questions. The first is to determine who is accountable for the parts of the prescribing journey and the second is whether accountability can be shared. Quite clearly, the prescribing decision was made by the nurse and so accountability for the decision would ultimately rest with the nurse prescriber. The nurse prescriber would show how local protocols had been followed and documentation was complete to support the prescribing decision. The nurse prescriber would need to demonstrate that they took the decision that rested within their own competency level.

The 'opening up of the prescription pad' was one of the defining moments when nursing had its freedom to act. However, with freedom to act is an acknowledgement of one's own limitations in knowing what is within your level of competency and, importantly, what is not. Nurses need to possess the skill of self-awareness in being aware of where their strengths lie and where they need to defer to specialist advice.

To put freedom to act in context, we can use the example of a nurse who prescribes morphine for substance misuse. The nurse will have a clear understanding of why they have prescribed morphine by taking the history. They will have diagnosed heroin addiction and will be aware of morphine as its substitute. The nurse would also be aware of how morphine raises QTc intervals in the cardiac rhythm and of the potentially fatal consequences. The nurse prescriber will be held accountable for the whole of the prescribing process including the outcome, both positive and untoward. With freedom to act is an understanding of why the intervention has been decided, and an acknowledgement that the nurse will be held accountable for that intervention.

It therefore brings into focus that nurse prescribers need to have knowledge on the condition to be treated, the risks of the treatment and how they can be managed. This is why nurses cannot defend a position of being unaccountable because they did not know about an intervention or the consequences of the intervention. If mental health nurse prescribers are unsure how to proceed in giving an intervention, then they should stop and seek advice of a knowledgeable colleague. Indeed, this very principle is enshrined in the legislation that governs prescribing when nurse prescribers should only work within their sphere of competence. The task is to ensure nurses are sufficiently self-aware to appreciate this point.

Freedom to act also implies authority to act. Authority for nurse prescribing is laid down clearly in supplementary prescribing in the form of a clinical management plan. In independent prescribing, authority to act is less clear apart from staying within the realms of the nurse's competency as defined by the nurse and the organisation. Organisations may wish to place limits on independent prescribing by specifying where nurses can prescribe through adherence to specific protocols.

Delegation

Delegation can be defined as the transfer of authority to a clinician not usually authorised to deliver an intervention to then follow the procedure. In order for nurse prescribers to be delegated too, nurses need to make sure that they have:

(1) knowledge and skills to deliver the intervention;
(2) access to the psychiatrist for on-going support;
(3) considered risks and benefits to the patient;
(4) safeguards to protect the patient;
(5) above all, the required competency to carry out the intervention.

Situations in which nurses may accept delegated responsibility are within the supplementary prescribing framework where medicines management is delegated from the psychiatrist to the nurse prescriber. Equally, a psychiatrist could delegate to an independent prescriber the care and treatment of an inpatient episode.

On a much simpler level, the nurse prescriber can delegate aspects of medicines management that although are not unauthorised interventions, they can be delivered with sufficient knowledge, skills and judgement by other nurses. However, as is often the case, medicines management is improperly delegated and is carried out below standards to that expected for people with mental health problems.

When delegation as a process is examined, it should usually include skill development through education and then an assessment of the competence of the clinician to deliver the intervention. Good practice is where aspects of delegated practice are covered in protocols and where the aspect of delegated medical practice is clearly described and fully understood by the person who is delegating the task and by the clinician who is accepting the delegation. It must be fully accepted by the nurse who agrees to the delegated task that they are competent to deliver the intervention, safely, and that their competence to deliver the intervention will be continuously reviewed. An example that can be used to illustrate this point is the delegated responsibility to follow the starting of clozapine for a patient with treatment resistant schizophrenia [drug licensed for schizophrenia (BNF 2008)]. Clozapine is a harmful drug that requires expertise in its side-effect management. It would be improper for a psych-iatrist to expect a nurse to manage the upward titration of clozapine without first checking their competency and knowledge regarding this drug.

Paternalism

Paternalism has been said to be justified when acting in the best interests of patients. However, patients are encouraged and now expect to exert choice in the clinical encounter. If nurse prescribers exert a paternalistic pattern of care, this would compromise choice. An obvious example is where a patient may be suited to a drug and this may fit their choice, but upon examination they may display symptoms of psychosis leading to disorganised thinking and behaviour. A nurse prescriber may wish to switch medication to exert a greater antipsychotic effect; however, this would compromise patient autonomy. The nurse would be acting in the patient's best interests but fails to communicate the decision or to collect the patient's view on the medication switch.

The nurse prescribing project is in real danger of misinterpreting the foundation for why nurses have been granted prescriptive privilege. Many policies have lamented from the start that nurse prescribing will increase access to medicines. The question to be considered is whether this is necessarily a good outcome for patients. For example, Granby (2007) noted that during 2005–2006, nonmedical prescribers prescribed 12.4 million products, and in the previous year, there was a 103% growth rate in the products supplied. In some quarters, these figures are celebrated as a success. There has been no inspection to make sure the products were appropriate or whether patients took more ownership in arranging their own medicinal requirements or alternative medical strategies.

The principle of paternalism is threatened by the desire of health services to be cost effective and to use the drug budget to meet the greatest need. New drugs come on to the market annually and nurse prescribers are keen to use these new drugs if they offer benefits in terms of efficacy. New drugs may come with a kinder side-effect profile and so offering greater tolerability. The problem is that new drugs tend to be more expensive. The choice over medication should be made in partnership with the patient, but the choice of drug is not always straightforward. The choice decision, however well intentioned, is strained to use the allocated drug budget to meet the greater good.

Beneficence

Two tensions exist within the principle of beneficence. The first is that we know that there are known side effects with antipsychotic medication; the second is that it is probable that when the patient takes the medication the nurse prescriber may well be bringing on untoward side effects. This is unavoidable for some patients. However, the flip side is that nurse prescribers may bring about untoward side effects simply because of poor prescribing practice; for example, polypharmacy in antipsychotic medication happens frequently in mental health services (NPSA 2006). For nurse prescribers to replicate this poor prescribing practice would be to carry on acting in a way which brings about harm to patients. Understandably, there are situations where patients require two different antipsychotic medications, particularly when switching from one to another. Poor prescribing practice would be for the prescriber to forget to cross off the previous medication.

Another area to do with beneficence is about iatrogenisis where the nurse-prescribing activity may bring about illnesses. For example, it is known that olanzapine and clozapine [drugs licensed for the treatment of schizophrenia (BNF 2008)] bring about weight gain for patients (Stahl 2006). Weight gain is strongly associated with glucose intolerance and high lipids in the blood, and overall forms a syndrome called metabolic syndrome (Sussman 2001).

Beneficence is an iterative process between the patient and the nurse prescriber where the nurse prescriber is continually adapting to increasing information about medicines and incorporating this into their prescribing practice. However, it is important that the nurse who is armed with all this knowledge does not fall into the trap of false notion that they know best, and lapses into paternalism. Nurse prescribers also have a duty not to cause harm to patients. It is known that medication does cause harmful effects, and for some people it can be fatal. Nurses may prevent harm occurring to patients by not only keeping up-to-date with information on medication but also being competent in their ability to prescribe medication.

Privilege

A nurse if given prescriptive authority could challenge the bedrock of what nurses and doctors do. However, the underbelly to this is that nurse prescribing is a privilege on a number of fronts. The first is about the type of society that we live in and the increasing drive to find the right 'pill'. We see evidence of society fracturing all the time and social distress being interpreted through a medical viewpoint. The pressure on nurses to prescribe is much more these days than it was in the olden days. One way to guard against this pressure is to regard prescribing as a privilege and not a right of acquiring passage for monetary or power reward.

The question for nurses to ask themselves is why legislation has been passed to enable them to prescribe. Arguments have been had on both sides trying to answer this question. Almost all revolve around perceived benefits for the patient, but they are hotly contested. Patients served by nurse prescribers want nurses to ensure they perceive their prescriptive authority as a privilege.

When nurses talk about prescribing, it is very easy for the discussion to be polarised into one of one gaining more power over the patient; power for the profession; power over other professions; and displacement of power from psychiatrists. What is lost in this professional tribalism is the sense that prescribing is a privilege, not a right or a prerequisite for the profession. When nurses start to use prescriptive authority and sign the prescription, the sense of accountability should be accompanied with the sense of privilege.

Knowledge and confidence

It is just unrealistic for nurses to acquire the breadth of knowledge to prescribe medication after they have completed the prescribing course. Even those nurses who work in single-disease areas where a limited number of drugs are prescribed require exposure to the realities of what can go wrong with drugs when prescribed incorrectly. If allowed to prescribe, nurses must be accompanied with humility in knowledge and acceptance that their psychiatric supervisors, provided they have been chosen selectively, have a vast reservoir of knowledge to be titrated over their prescribing career.

The opposite to this argument however is the lack of confidence to prescribe. This is a problem discussed previously in this book and is equally destroying the act of prescribing as being dangerously unaware of knowledge about medication. The Nursing & Midwifery Council (2006) is clear in that nurses are responsible for conducting themselves within their scope of competency and to use the knowledge appropriately. Knowledge and confidence to prescribe go hand in hand for effective prescribing practice.

Mental Health Act

When patients are admitted into hospital, it is conceivable that their admission or continued admission may be through the Mental Health Act (DoH 2008b). Patients who are detained under the Mental Health Act (DoH 2008b) should not be denied access to nurses who can prescribe medication. As demonstrated through the practical implementation of nurse prescribing, patients can receive a more efficient and effective monitoring and review of medication, targeted education and interventions to support concordance. When the guidance on the implementation of supplementary prescribing is examined, it suggests that the patient should enter into the prescribing relationship voluntarily and consent to the treatment being offered to them (DoH 2003). A patient may not give their consent for the wider treatment plan for their mental disorder (e.g. for being admitted into hospital), but the patient may give consent for the prescription of medication. In this regard, it seems justifiable that the patient may consent to nurse prescribing.

To illustrate this point, one can consider a patient who has been detained under Section 3 of the Mental Health Act (DoH 2008b). The patient may consent to the nurse being their supplementary prescriber for the first 3 months of the treatment. If after 3 months, continued treatment is still required under detention, the psychiatrist would complete Form 38 and specify the drugs listed on the clinical management plan. Form 38 and the clinical management plan are then stapled to the inpatient treatment card.

Significantly, it must be remembered that patients who are detained in hospital should not be discriminated against in terms of expert interventions that can arise through mental health nurse prescribing.

Capacity and consent

One of the biggest legal threats that the nurse prescribers may experience is 'trespass to the person'. This is interpreted as assault and battery. It is important that the nurse prescriber seeks and gains the patient's consent for interventions that are to be delivered. The nurse can do this by approaching the patient at the earliest opportunity to discuss treatment options. Nurses will need to take account of the patient's illness and to consider whether the condition affects the patient's capacity to make a decision about their care. The obvious example here is of the patient with advanced-stage dementia who is unable to take in information. Other patients may be so psychotic that they do not understand what the nurse prescriber is saying to them about their treatment. In this respect, the patient may not be able to give informed consent to the nurse being a prescriber or to accepting the medication.

Nurses need to ensure they give patients sufficient information in a format that is accessible. Nurse prescribers may wish to do this in conjunction with the patient's family or carer to aid understanding. As far as possible, nurses need to use language that is free from medical jargon that alienates patients.

There are patients who have severe dementia and may not understand that you are a nurse acting in their best interests by prescribing diazepam to control arousal. How can the nurse prescribe medication in these situations without assessing the patient's capacity to consent to treatment? Would it be legal for the nurse to prescribe medication in the best interests of the patient? New legislation helps to define the stages for assessing capacity under the Mental Capacity Act (2005).

Nurse prescribing is a consensual activity. It requires a dialogue with the patient where the condition to be treated and medicines to be used are explained. For nurse prescribing, the patient's consent is always required. The case study above illustrates the dilemma that nurse prescribers face when patients begin to loose understanding about treatment options put before them. It would be important for the nurse prescriber to ensure that the consent to

> **Case Study**
>
> Jim is 64 and has been suffering from moderate short-term memory loss for 2 years. He has been assessed in the memory clinic and deemed suitable for the antidementia drug Aricept [licensed for the treatment of dementia (BNF 2008)]. Julie is assigned to be his care coordinator and to prescribe the drug. When Julie explains the drug treatment, Jim does not show evidence that he understands the treatment being offered to him. Jim also does not understand that Julie will be acting as his independent nurse prescriber.

treatment protocols are being followed and that information relating to this process is clearly documented. Some patients may have capacity for 1 week, and for it to diminish some times later. Nurses may wish to discuss advanced treatment directives when the patient lacks capacity. Advanced directives need to be clearly documented and accessible to the care team (DoH 2008a).

Pharmaceutical industry

The pharmaceutical industry is part and parcel of health care in the UK. They are an important driver for developing new technologies. Patients do benefit from the medicines they take. Nurses also benefit from education and training, not only on drugs advocated by the particular company but also on nonpromotional workshop topics. However, the pharmaceutical industry will find out who is qualified to prescribe medication and target them as a potential customer.

The obvious temptation that exists with the pharmaceutical industry is their immense wealth to influence prescribers across all disciplines. Evidence does show that when drug representatives target a drug in a particular area, drug sales go up. In 1997, the industry spent just over £500m to promote their drugs in the UK. A United States report noted that pharmaceutical companies spend roughly twice as much on marketing [30%] than it did on research [12%] (Public Citizen 2001). Therefore, the pharmaceutical industry is able to successfully influence to meet its ends. The message here is that nurse prescribers need to accept the pharmaceutical industry as a major partner in care but to seriously question any evidence that is produced by them to support their product.

Ethically, nurses must not put themselves forward in promoting a drug without first putting forward a declaration of interest. Organisations should also maintain a register to record when health employees undertake work for the pharmaceutical industry. Nurses need to find out about this register and how to use it to protect themselves against unfair criticism if they are employed to carry out work for the pharmaceutical industry.

An often quoted criticism of nurses is that they are more susceptible and gullible to ill effects of drug company sales staff. One explanation may be the positive strokes nurses receive from their organisation compared to doctors, or what they perceive doctors to receive compared to themselves. The pharmaceutical industry will be able to pick up on these cues and readily supply complements to nursing staff on the positive effects they have on patient care. The bottom line is that nurses need to learn how to negotiate with pharmaceutical representatives so that they can extract their information and support needs without necessarily being drawn into the specific product. Nurse prescribers need to own the responsibility to scrutinise information and to use this information wisely.

One way to disentangle the perceived and actual effect pharmaceutical industry has on nurse prescribers would be to up front with patients about contact you have had with drug representatives or any sponsorship work carried out for the company. Transparency between the prescriber and the patient is important, and this would be one way to bring this about.

A general point here needs to be made about the ability of nurses to approach the evidence base with a degree of critical awareness. Drug companies will be happy to give what appear to be respectable 'gold standard' research data from high-ranking journals. Evidence is portrayed in such a way that leaves the naive clinician with a view that wonders why not all patients are prescribed a certain drug. A simple fact is that of all trial data for people with schizophrenia, patients who have substance misuse, suicidal behaviour and disruptive behaviour would be excluded (Thornley & Adams 2000). Many of our patients do not fit these criteria, so extrapolation to every day services is near enough impossible.

Conclusion

The ethical and professional regulation for nurse prescribing is laid down by the Nursing & Midwifery Council (2006), and nurse prescribers are bound by the code of conduct. Nurses must find their own moral compass within the boundaries laid down and remember the privilege they have been given when accorded the responsibilities of being a nurse prescriber.

The ethical and professional regulation has no legal status because it only regulates conduct. However, if the nurse is found to have operated outside of their code of conduct, this can be used as evidence in a civil breach of duty or criminal prosecution. Nurses are individually accountable to the Nursing & Midwifery Council (2006). Nurses must ensure that they prescribe within the limits of their competency in order for them to be protected from legal liability claims in the advent of untoward incidents. Nurses must also be mindful to think what their employing organisation has carried out to protect themselves and the nurse prescriber in the event of an untoward incident. It would be strongly advised for nurse prescribers to work to a protocol that governs what area of practice the nurse prescriber intends to practice in and what medicines they intend to use.

In considering the legal issues behind nurse prescribing, nurses must not be tempted to abandon the journey that they have started. It would be easy to forgive those nurses who decide that the risks are too high for them to be a nurse prescriber given the legal precedents that have been laid before them. However, it is equally important to recognise that case law is in place to protect them.

Chapter 11
Future challenges for nurse prescribers

Introduction

This book has been about unleashing and delivering the potential of nurse prescribing. It has set out the challenges and drivers for the future and highlights the fundamental issues that need to be addressed. Perhaps most important, and which strikes at the core value of nursing, is to enable nurses to care and treat patients in a person-centred way. Sometimes the human touch of what is psychiatric nursing can become lost in the excitement of nurse prescribing. Whilst acknowledging that nursing has to change, it is important that the core values remain in tact.

There is still a lack of clarity about the future workforce planning and emerging roles. However, it is inevitable that new roles and responsibilities will all require some form of prescriptive authority. Safety, regulation and ongoing training demand continuous adaptation to meet the ever-increasing requirement for safer services.

The advancement of science will bring new technologies to the fore. Nurse prescribers will interface with the new communication and information technologies to gain further knowledge. Bringing this information resource closer to the patient decision-making juncture may improve the quality of the prescribing advice given to patients. All will assist in the decision-making process and for nurse prescribing to be safe. Safe services should be the main objective when nurse prescribing is introduced.

Many of the areas where mental health nurses work offer potential for the development of nonmedical prescribing. Future research needs to consider how the role of a nurse prescriber adds something different to the health encounter or whether it simply replicates what is already there, in terms of junior and consultant psychiatrists. Nurses who prescribe medication need to connect with what patients want from the encounter.

Increased patient choice and involvement

People who use these services now present with needs different from those they did 30 years ago. Patients want control over their health care and to influence how it is delivered, particularly for medicines management (National Prescribing Centre 2008). Moreover, they wish to have a personal service where they are not passed from pillar to post to receive treatment and care. Health care in the future will need to respond to an agenda where consumer experience is high.

Wanless (2002) came to the conclusion that the NHS is structured around acute provision with little emphasis on health promotion and self-promotion of health. However, British society is changing; patients are now more likely to look at the effects of taking medication and then go and ask for it from their general practitioner or nurse prescriber.

Patients very often express a wish about how they want to be treated, although services do not always hear the language. Health teams have flirted with techniques to address concordance and persuade people to turn up for appointments. We have popularly described this as the choice agenda but it is really an ever-increasing consciousness of the public to the deep-seated institutional and professional disregard for patient involvement. We accept that not all clinicians or patients will support this new way of thinking, but people must be bold to embrace a more balanced way of engaging with patients. Nurse prescribers must be in the vanguard of this development, ready and waiting to serve the public.

Health care needs to change from being an acute focused service and take on wider determinants of health such as health promotion, illness prevention and management of long-term conditions. Nurses will need to have a broader range of skills to meet the different needs of our patients. For example, helping an increasingly older population to remain well and to self-manage their conditions at home. This is against a context where one in four people suffer a lifetime prevalence of depression. This is why the next-generation nurse prescribers will need to be flexible and adaptable to work across different care and home environments. The centre of gravity will shift to working more with people closer to home hence the need for nurses to have prescriptive authority that is not tied to institutional practices.

The UK government and service user organisations illuminate patients' wish for greater say in how health care is delivered. Patients want shared decision making in health care and up-to-date information. They also want their health care to be person centred with fewer waiting times and onward referral. A question that revolves around all our developments for health care is whether nurse prescribing will make any difference to the outcomes of care.

Positions in society are changing and the public is becoming cynical about healthcare delivery. However, the societal position of doctors is highly cherished and patients still want to see their doctor. Patients are critical of system changes in accessing primary care, principally because they have a relationship with their own general practitioner. However, patients are starting to accept more nonmedical prescribers and the status of nurse prescribers was not their main concern (Berry *et al.* 2006).

Nurse prescribing will provide greater opportunities for patients to gain access to medication as a treatment option. However, is this a good outcome for patients? Inadvertently, nurse prescribing may actually push up the medicalisation of mental illness and the increasing number of drugs that are being prescribed in practice. This is not a good outcome for nurse prescribing. Much emphasis has been placed on alternatives to drug treatments that patients may choose.

The whole point of nurse prescribing is to enable patients to exercise their choices in the type of clinician or intervention or environment in which they wish to be treated. Choice obviously infers that there is a suitable range of options for how treatment can be delivered.

Connecting the future labour market to service improvement

The way nurses work today reflects the preoccupations and aspirations of a workforce, largely from the post-war baby boom and a group of people born between 1965 and 1985. New technologies, changing consumer expectations, changes to professional and regulatory frameworks drive the need to modernise the workforce. Within most quarters, it is accepted that the workforce needs to change to meet the needs of the population. Fundamental to these changes are role adaptation to think much more laterally about the place of work and how nurses can work across service settings in managing patient care (Jones *et al.* 2005).

The record levels of NHS investment over the last decade are unlikely to be repeated. The increased demand for services will need to be met by making the current staff more productive. The development of the nursing workforce to undertake prescribing activity is a key driver to deliver a modernised service. Prescribing needs to be structured so that different levels of nurses can practise a level of prescribing. Education and professional regulations need to be continually updated to take account of advanced practice roles that will emerge in the future.

The current framework for training nurses to use prescriptive authority is inflexible. We also have evidence of a number of reasons why nurses don't use their new authority when trained. There is considerable scope to introduce the principles of medicines management and the prescription of a limited number of drugs at the preregistration level. This will help to broaden the concept of nursing responsibilities for medicines management. The introduction of nurse prescribing at the preregistration level also cements the concept of nurse prescribing being a competency-based activity that develops with experience and further training.

A criticism levelled at nurse prescribing is that you are getting doctors on the cheap (Jones 2008). In other words, nurses are carrying out tasks once traditionally undertaken by doctors, such as diagnosis and prescribing medication. However, is nurse prescribing really that cheap? Doctors may arrive at a diagnosis and treatment plan far quicker than nursing staff and communicate this to patients. The caveat to this, however, is that patients are critical of the quality of the information coming from medical staff. Doctors may be more productive, even though they are more expensive. Another example that undermines the 'doctors on the cheap' perspective is the position of junior doctors. To employ a nurse who can prescribe independently would be far more expensive than to employ a junior doctor.

Factors to consider for the preparation of nurse practitioners who can prescribe, for example, include the cost of further education, supervision costs, infrastructure from within and outside the health sector and most importantly lost hours through staff being on additional training (Curtis & Netten 2007). A positive attribute of nurse prescribing is that the prescriber, compared to the general practitioner, spends longer time carrying out the intervention with the patient. Horrocks *et al.* (2002) also found this with nurse practitioners, but one could argue that care by general practitioners is more efficient because more patients are seen. A recent randomised controlled trial found that adding nurse practitioners to a general practice did not lessen the workload of general practitioners (Laurant *et al.* 2004). This dents the argument that adding in nurses with extended skills is about substituting the role of doctors because, in fact, the agenda is about enhancing the quality of care.

Role change and substitution from medical staff to nurses have been studied extensively in the UK. The development of advanced nurse practitioner posts is pertinent to the debate on changing roles. Buchan & Calman (2005) examined skill mix from the perspective of a number of European states and the USA and confirmed skill shortages within healthcare teams to be the main driver for the introduction of the advanced nurse practitioner role. Particularly to the UK, policy changes such as the effects of the European Working Time Directive and the reform of nursing careers have also been influential (DoH 2006e, 2007a,b). These changes should be viewed in a positive light so that the quality of the patient experience becomes the *raison d'être* of service development.

A question frequently asked by nurses and doctors is whether nurse prescribers, with their added skills, will replace psychiatrists. The answer is firmly no. To agree with this statement misses the essence of what nurse prescribers will do in the future. Our vision for the future is that nurse prescribers will complement the existing staff group skills. You are more likely to find nurses managing patients who do not need to be seen by psychiatrists. This does not mean removing doctors from the team of healthcare practitioners. In contrast, psychiatrists are more likely to see the sickest patients more often. The upshot of this is that role substitution is not as simple as saying that nurses can replace doctors or aspects of their work. There is also a lack of studies that comprehensively look at the economic implications of substituting one cheaper profession for another. This will be a drawback on persuading medical staff to freely give up aspects of their role in the absence of evidence. Psychiatrists have been fairly derisory towards the concept of distributed responsibility epitomised in new ways of working (Gee 2007; Craddock *et al.* 2008).

In the future, will we see a situation where health care will be in crisis because the right number of professionals is not available? The population is certainly rising and the public health agenda of a growing elderly population is making health care complex. The population is also becoming more diverse where health inequalities will arise in pockets of underserved communities. The question is whether nurse prescribers will meet this need, which adds quality and safety to the intervention.

Nurses have been adept at evolving and taking on new roles and skills. The government drive to increase the workforce has been most successful with the nursing profession. Nurses pride themselves on delivering health targets. Nurses are working in different settings and new teams and developing partnerships with patients based on choice and user involvement. It is in this context that professional boundaries become blurred. However, for nurse prescribing to be successfully introduced into the 'psych' of mental health nurses, nurses will need to broaden their technical skill set.

The nursing workforce has many strengths in that it is adaptable and can be moulded to suit care environments such as hospitals, the diverse array of community services and the various specialist clinic environments. It is too early to say how nurse prescribing will change the workforce; however, it is reasonable to conclude that the legislation allowing nurses to prescribe medication helps oil the wheels of change, so that the workforce can modernise and take on work and extend their boundaries of influence over patient care. Questions over what a qualified nurse is required to do in different care environments is again outside the scope of this book, but there is a very clear direction that nurses will take on aspects of work that require diagnostic abilities, treatment formulation and care management roles.

Prescriptive authority will help the workforce to become more flexible because it enables those professions that are the highest skilled in their diagnosis and treatment to take on more appropriate work streams. Nurse prescribing also brings into focus the range of skills held by qualified nurses and what is actually expected from a qualified nurse. We may actually see a reduction in the number of qualified nurses, with their work carried out by a more diverse array of nonprofessionally aligned workers. With this migration, it seems reasonable to conclude that a larger number of specialist nurses will emerge.

Nurse prescribing will not only allow the opportunity for flexible clinicians but also bring to life the concept of flexible teams. Nurse prescribing is not an isolated intervention. Nurse prescribing occurs as part of a wider team where a skill set is required that allows the nurse to mould the culture of the team and, in turn, the culture of the team to mould the way of working of the nurse prescriber. Nurse prescribing requires flexible teams and flexible ways of thinking about how resources will be deployed. However, we do need to find out what will sustain and hold back the whole notion of flexible teams.

Pharmacists are valuable members of the healthcare team, but for mental health, the number is very small. They are eligible to be trained as supplementary and independent prescribers, and in some trusts, pharmacists undertake this role. However, it seems a better use of this highly specialised resource, for the time that phamacists would spend prescribing to be spent on supervision with nursing staff. Simple strategies to bring this about may be including mental health pharmacists in support groups for nurses, setting up supervision sessions and teaching sessions.

Simply adding in more nurses who can prescribe medication will allow greater capacity within the service. Independent prescribing requires the nurse to be able to take a history, develop formulations, plan treatments and so take on some of the tasks previously undertaken by junior medical staff and consultant psychiatrists. The question that needs to be answered is whether the services really needs nurses to carry out this work and whether patients actually want to be seen by a nurse prescriber or a doctor, no matter how junior that doctor may be. One also needs to ask about the quality of the diagnosis and formulation and whether this meets acceptable standards of governance within this increasingly risk containment NHS culture.

Nursing is being put forward as a competency-based profession across all areas and domains of work. The intention is not to produce nurses who would become an expert but those who are required by the service. In this situation, nurses would become specialised and those nurses with advanced skills would manage patients with the most complex needs. Nursing would occupy all strands of health care, delivering care at one end of the spectrum and diagnostics and treatment at the other end. No particular value judgement is meant by placing care and treatment on this continuum.

It stands to reason that if you have appropriately trained nursing staff who can prescribe medication as part of their skill set and then deploy this workforce appropriately, patients would then have improved access to advice and service. The benefits and drawbacks of specialising nursing staff is beyond the scope of this book; however, nurses who are trained and work in specialist fields are likely to develop high levels of expertise in the management of the condition. This expertise is likely to go beyond the generic expertise held by general practitioners. Patient safety somehow seems more assured by nurses who work in specialist teams and would be an obvious area for development.

How do we prepare our staff for the role?

A pressing concern for researchers and clinicians is the effectiveness and efficiency of the prescribing training programme for nurses from different specialties (Hemingway & Davies 2005). It is quite possible that the concerns over nurse prescribing, particularly independent prescriptive authority, will be addressed through 'top-up' training and support (Skingsley *et al.* 2006). However, one must question whether this piece meal approach makes best use of staff time or assures quality. In order for nurse prescribing to advance with confidence, concerns about the length, depth and variability of the current methods of training nurses to prescribe must be addressed (Banning 2004; Bradley *et al.* 2006). Nurse education also needs to support system change so that new roles incumbent with nurse prescribing can be put into practice.

In order for this to take place, nursing registration should be conducted at graduate levels. National quality standards should be in place to protect the public's safety. Nurses must be trained to think within a competency framework where they can develop the ability to learn and acquire knowledge through their experiences. In order for them to do this, they must be able to take decisions based on evidence and to take independent action. This may then help to build a bridge that is commonplace nowadays between how doctors and nurses think.

Nurse education should be viewed as a continuous career and lifelong learning experience. Nurse prescribing demands a conceptual and technical adaptation to diagnostics and therapeutics. The regulatory milestones that have been proposed so far are helpful, but these are to be extended as nurses take on more advanced roles. Contributors towards this unclear alignment are the education providers, service leaders and commissioners.

A major issue for nurse-prescribing training is the wastage through people not practising upon qualification. Further studies needs to be carried out to make selection processes more effective. Part of the problem is to fully understand the gaps in workforce planning and a failure to understand the clinical scenarios where nurse prescribing would be effective.

Nurse prescribers will require a set of new skills to enable them to work within their own clinical specialties. These skills will become more advanced when they take on independent prescribing responsibilities. Chapters 5–8 provide much of the content for consideration by nurse prescribers as they enter the world of delivering diagnostics and treatment. Table 11.1 recaps the major education and training components for mental health nurses.

Some organisations are preparing nurses with particular modules such as diagnostic skills and medication management skills. Scope certainly exists for trusts and universities to develop mental health-specific training packages. The next step is accreditation.

A very positive picture of how nurse prescribing can work in practice has been presented. However, we must acknowledge that not all nurses welcome the increased responsibility and workload (Nolan *et al.* 2001) and some nurses

Table 11.1 Areas for training and development to enable nurses to practise safely and within expected competency

History, mental state examination and diagnosis	Bedrock of supplementary and independent prescribing
Formulate and implement treatment plan	Team-based prescribing and how to work to a distributed care model arrangement
Medication management	Knowledge of tools and techniques to support patients in their medication management
Patient education and health promotion	Knowledge of how patients can be supported to manage their health
Referral to psychiatrists when competency is breached	Clear training in working within competency and use of competency frameworks (National Prescribing Centre 2004)
Medical treatment and referral pathways for coexisting medical conditions	Knowledge of coexisting medical conditions that occur frequently with psychiatric disorders

Table 11.2 Dimension of change for nurse prescribers

Coming from	Changing to
Medical decision making where psychiatrists take decisions	Nurse-led care and nurses managing episodes of care within their competency
Unclear roles for prescribers	Job adverts that have nurse prescribing as essential for the post
Fragmented educational preparation	Fully developed courses that enable nurses to prescribe medication as part of an extended role
Piece meal competency learned on the job	A seal of competency that assures prescribing safety along with other key skills such as diagnostics
Nurse prescribers working in the NHS	Nurse prescribers setting up entrepreneurial schemes to meet consumer needs

fear the increased accountability that will follow (Bradley *et al.* 2005). However, nurse prescribing is a growing activity. This is only the start of a long development process. A clear strategy for nurse prescribing must be to decide how we take the public, the service and the professions with us on this journey. The nursing profession is changing within a healthcare environment that is constantly shifting. Table 11.2 looks at a number of dimensions where the culture of nursing is shifting towards greater accountability.

Although symptomatic of the changing direction of health care and nurse prescribing, we have seen a plethora of new titles, new roles and different types of services. This has caused tension within the profession, and certainly, there has been some tidying up of the types of prescribing titles. We are about to embark on having responsible clinicians under the reformed Mental Health Act (DoH 2008b). It will be interesting to see how this role develops a sense of permanency and role expectation and how the public responds to this role. Policy documents such as modernising nursing careers (DoH 2006e), workforce reviews (DoH 2008c) and regulatory documents by the Nursing & Midwifery Council (2006, 2007) have at their heart protection of the public, as redefined nurses take on autonomous forms of practice. 'Tomorrow's clinicians' (DoH 2008c, page 8) are the aspirations for nurse prescribers.

Be political to affect implementation

Nurse prescribing has moved on considerably from the early work set out by Julia Cumberlidge in the early 1980s. Diffusion of these new skills into the healthcare setting has at best been patchy and some areas of nursing have been more successful than others in their implementation strategy.

However, the opportunities for implementation are numerous across our healthcare system. None of the barriers to change are insurmountable. The solutions discussed are achievable within the existing resources. Chapter 4 reviewed in detail how nurse prescribers can penetrate and influence key decision makers in organisations. The challenge is for nurse prescribers, psychiatrists and service planners to be open minded about how the nurse-prescribing resource can be best utilised and be willing to take positive risks in order to achieve the benefits that will flow.

Successful implementation of nurse prescribing is about effective teamwork and a strategic vision being articulated by and to the organisation. There are numerous reports that have helped to set the direction and approach that organisations and individuals should take (National Prescribing Centre 2005a; DoH 2008d). These reports have provided a structured way of helping teams and individuals to reflect on the current and future capabilities of both themselves and the organisation to help implement nurse prescribing.

There are encouraging signals that nurse prescribing is beginning to work; however the reality is that it is occurring only in a minority of trusts. This book will help individuals and organisations to make sure that nurse prescribing takes place in more organisations and is embedded into the culture of care. Major challenges will continue to emerge with independent prescriptive authority.

It is vital that nurses at all levels feel confidant and supported when they are carrying out nurse prescribing. The two sources of support are from their professional body and their organisation. The Nursing & Midwifery Council (2006) has developed a clear ethical framework that will guide nurse prescribers certainly for the next few years. However, the clinical landscape is changing constantly. New roles are emerging as more care becomes devolved quite rightly from medical staff and where nurses can work in areas of work that successfully meets the needs of patients.

Organisations also need to support nurse prescribers. Organisations by their very nature are conservative and limiting in terms of what they allow nurses to do. Nurse prescribers need to understand the position of clinical governance and vicarious liability and to make sure that the practices that they wish to use are supported by evidence and have been widely consulted upon. Nurse prescribers also need to make sure that the governance arrangements surrounding their practice have been carefully considered so that the safety of patients remains paramount at all times. If nurses consider these main points, then organisational resistance to nurse prescribing may be lessened.

Nurse prescribing is a central plank in planning and sustaining the workforce across the whole range of mental health services. Nurse prescribing is not just about the giving of pills. Role change and new ways of working are challenged. What is clear from the research on nurse prescribing is that implementation of this approach cannot occur in a vacuum. Nurse prescribing requires a whole system change that incorporates a review of traditional roles and expectations and also incorporates the choice agenda.

The position taken throughout this book is that nurse prescribing is an intervention that has come about as the profession of nursing has come of age. The advancement of medical procedures, and the ability to understand how procedures work, has helped to teach these procedures to nurses. Nurses are lesser qualified than doctors but are able practitioners to deliver interventions safely to certain groups of patients. In other words, it is a logical extension of what some nurses should be doing to meet the needs of patients. This is a laudable logical conclusion. Indeed there are many examples of roles and tasks undertaken by junior and senior medical staff that are now delivered competently by nursing staff.

Many platitudes are used to distinguish nursing from medicine, such as nursing being a unique person-centred approach, holistic in its intent with a strong underbelly of care. Some have suggested that the government has introduced nurse prescribing as a political manoeuvre to fill in the gaps created by the shortage of doctors and ultimately as a cost-cutting exercise (Horton 1992). Perhaps the real reason is to offer patients different access points to the service to challenge the bedrock of medical hegemony. If this line of argument is accepted, then the political objectives will indeed be met. However, this aside, nurses may well exert greater political influence by working in a way that is ethically different from that of other prescribers. Chapter 10 has introduced the reader to some of the main ethical principles, and when nurses articulate an ethical way of working through their practice, patients may start to prefer this way of working.

Patient safety

Patient safety is paramount to our desire to deliver effective care. Nurse-prescribing policy has been at pains to highlight the importance of safety (DoH 2006b). However, further development of the policy is required to point out clear governance structures and regulatory frameworks. A clear example of lax control is the progression of nurses from supplementary to independent prescriptive authority. The government policy has placed the responsibility on the employing organisations to ensure nurses work within their area of competency (DoH 2006b). It also places responsibility on practitioners for staying within their areas of competence.

The bottom line is that nurse prescribing needs to be safe for patients. Studies need to cover whether nurses prescribe the best medication for patients and whether the training and support is in place for this to occur consistently. It is also required to identify what new risks that nonmedical prescribing introduces into health care and how they can be managed.

Accountability for care is also becoming more important as the variable standards are being questioned and clinicians being brought to account. Nurses therefore need to be clear that they act only within their competency and refer to their supervisor when this competency has been reached. Not many studies have been carried out in this area and it remains to be seen how confident and willing nurses would be in consulting on areas outside their competency range.

Robust governance is essential for nurse prescribing. If nurse prescribing is audited as an isolated practice, it may not reveal discrepancies against usual practice within the organisation. Patient safety can be further assured by annual audits of all nurse prescribers within the organisation.

The function of being a nurse prescriber should be located within a particular job title such as a nurse consultant or nurse practitioner. Junior staff nurses and community nurses may also carry out a prescribing role within their area of competency. Standardisation of roles and responsibilities needs to take place so that consistency is applied across the nurse prescriber role. This should help to clear up the confusion over role titles.

However, it is not just the title that is confusing; the scope of practice carried out by different specialists is also not clear. Inadvertently, the current situation does not protect the public, as they cannot be assured of what further training nurses have received or their scope of practice. The nurse prescribing qualification does not assure patients of an educationally prepared scope of competency. A nurse prescriber must not be seen as a role descriptor but function as part of a job role.

A final word must be said about continuous professional development, supervision and competency, which are required for safe nurse prescribing, although when questioned, 84% of nurse prescribers felt they required further support for professional development opportunities (National Prescribing Centre 2005c). Otway (2002) found that nurse prescribers were not engaging with supervision programmes even though this is essential for safe prescribing. The Nursing & Midwifery Council (2006, 2007) has also laid down unambiguous statements for nurse prescribers to practice within a safe and legal framework in terms of competency.

Organisations have a part to play in ensuring nurses not only have access to training and development but also abide by strict competency frameworks. Running through this book has been the central role of psychiatrists in assuring competency and further developing competency to practice. Organisations have developed user-friendly competency frameworks not only for actual skills in prescribing (National Prescribing Centre 2003) but also for shared decision making with patients (National Prescribing Centre 2007), and these should be developed further within local services. The central point being made here is that nurses are accountable for their practice and nurse prescribing defines the scope of practice even further. The nursing profession will require ongoing monitoring on its journey in managing the complexity of disease groups. As Chapter 1 made it clear, the entwined relationship between nurses and psychiatrists is replicated and strengthened with nurse prescribing. This should be celebrated as we move forward into the 21st century.

Conclusion

Mental health nurses in the UK work in a variety of roles and service settings. They are the largest professional group in health care and this is their strength to exert a change in how patients receive care and treatment. Key to this change is to ensure nurses meet the needs of patients. Central to this is the role of nurse prescribing so that patients can receive more of the service component from a provider without onward referral. However, it is only the start of the journey for nurse prescribing. Research and anecdotal accounts report hampering and sustaining factors across organisational, education and professional domains. Many of these can be overcome to enable nurse prescribing to succeed.

The key messages contained in this book revolve around safe effective services delivered by appropriately skilled and knowledgeable practitioners. Nurses must ensure that they do not abandon their core values of human partnership when they take on prescribing responsibilities.

It was stated at the beginning of this book that nurse prescribing is not just about giving medication to patients. Nurses have carried out this function de facto since medication was first developed. Also rejected is the accusation that nurse prescribing is an abandonment of core nursing skills. The key message is about patient partnership and using this partnership to bring about improved patient outcomes in areas such as symptom management, better physical health and preservation of life. Nurse prescribers will have tremendous potential to deliver this agenda and will certainly take its place as one of the modern advances of the nursing profession.

References

Age Concern (2008). The Age Agenda Conference 2008. Age Concern England, London. Accessed at: http://www.ageconcern.org.uk/AgeConcern/3D21CD1299E04A97AAB7B91EF45 F5D16.asp

Allsop A., Brooks L., Bufton L., Carr C., Courtney Y., Dale C., Pittard S., & Thomas C. (2005). Supplementary prescribing in mental health and learning disabilities. Nursing Standard 19(30), 54–58.

An Bord Altranais (2005). Review of Nurses and Midwives in the Prescribing and Administration of Medicinal Products. ABA, Dublin.

Anderson P. & Baumberg B. (2006). Alcohol in Europe: A Public Health Perspective. Institute of Alcohol Studies, London.

Andreasen N.C. & Carpenter W.T. (1993). Diagnosis and classification of schizophrenia. Schizophrenia Bulletin 19, 199–214.

Angermeyer M.C., Boitz K. & Loffler W. (1999). Attitude of family to clozapine. Psychiatric Praxis 26, 181–187.

Appleby L. (2006). Avoidable Deaths. The University of Manchester, Manchester.

Assmann G., Schulte H., von Eckardstein A. & Huang Y. (1996). High-density lipoprotein cholesterol as a predictor of coronary heart disease risk. The PROCAM experience and pathophysiological implications for reverse cholesterol transport. Atherosclerosis 124(Suppl), S11–S20.

Audit Commission (2001). A spoonful of sugar – medicines management in NHS hospitals. Accessed at: http://www.audit-commission.gov.uk

Avery J.A. & Pringle M. (2005). Extended prescribing by UK nurses and pharmacists. British Medical Journal 331(7526), 1154–1155.

Babiker I.E. (1986). Non-compliance in schizophrenia. Psychiatric Developments 4, 329–337.

Bailey K. (1999). Framework for prescriptive practice (Chapter 13). In: C. Shea, L. Pelletier, E. Poster, G. Stuart & M. Verhey (Eds.). Advanced Practice Nursing in Psychiatric and Mental Health Care. Mosby, New York.

Baker A., Boggs T.G. & Lewin T.J. (2001). Randomized controlled trial of brief cognitive-behavioural interventions among regular users of amphetamine. Addiction 96(9), 1279–1287.

Baker J.A., Lovell K., Harris N. & Campbell M. (2007). Multidisciplinary consensus of best practice for pro re nata (PRN) psychotropic medications within acute mental health settings: a Delphi study. Journal of Psychiatric and Mental Health Nursing 14, 478–484.

Banning M. (2004). Nurse prescribing, nurse education and related research in the United Kingdom: a review of the literature. Nurse Education Today 24, 420–427.

Barcroft S. (2005). Nurse prescribing in substance misuse. Accessed at: http://www.nta.nhs.uk/publications/documents/nta_nurse_prescribing_in_substance_misuse_may_2005.pdf

Barker P.J., Jackson S. & Stevenson C. (1999). The need for psychiatric nursing: towards a multidimensional theory of caring. Nursing Inquiry 6(2), 103–111.

Barker P.J. & Walker L. (2000). Nurses' perceptions of multidisciplinary teamwork in acute psychiatric settings. Journal of Psychiatric and Mental Health Nursing 7, 539–546.

Barlow M., Majorrian K. & Jones M. (2008). Nurse prescribing in an Alzheimer's disease service: a reflective account. Mental Health Practice 11, 32–35.

Barnes T.R.E. (1989). A rating scale for drug-induced akathisia, British Journal of Psychiatry 154, 672—676.

Bazire S. (2007). Psychotropic Drug Directory. Fivepin, Wiltshire.

Beattie A. (1995). War and peace amongst the health tribes. In: K. Soothill, L. Mackay & C. Webb (Eds.). Interpersonal relations in health care. Edward Arnold, London.

Beck A., Steer R. & Brown G. (1987). Beck Depression Inventory 2. The Psychological Corporation, San Antonio.

Bedi N., Chilvers C., Churchill R., et al. (2000). Assessing effectiveness of treatment of depression in primary care. Partially randomised preference trial. British Journal of Psychiatry 177, 312–318.

Bennett J., Done J. & Hunt B. (1995). Assessing the side effects of antipsychotic drugs: a survey of CPN practice. Journal of Psychiatric and Mental Health Nursing 2, 177–182.

Benson K.L. (2006) Psychiatric Clinics North America 26, 1033–45.

Berger G.E., Proffitt T. & Wood S. (2004). Ethyl-eicosapentaenoic acid supplementation in early psychosis: a double-blind randomised placebo-controlled add on study in 80 drug naïve first episode psychosis patients. International Journal of Neuropsychopharmacology 8(1), S422.

Berry D., Courtenay M. & Bersellini E. (2006). Attitudes towards, and information needs in relation to, supplementary nurse prescribing in the UK: an empirical study. Journal of Clinical Nursing 15(1), 22–28.

Blenkinsopp A., Bond C., Britten N., et al. (1997). From compliance to concordance: achieving shared goals in medicine taking. A working party report. Royal Pharmaceutical Society of Great Britain, London.

Blenkiron P. (1998). Referral to a psychiatric clinic: what do patients expect? International Journal of Health Care Quality Assurance 11, 188–192.

Bowles N. & Jones A. (2005). Whole systems working and acute inpatient psychiatry: an exploratory study. Journal of Psychiatric and Mental Health Nursing 12, 283–289.

Bradley E., Campbell P. & Nolan P. (2005). Nurse prescribers: who are they and how do they perceive their role? Journal of Advanced Nursing 51(5), 439–448.

Bradley E., Blackshaw C. & Nolan P. (2006). Nurse lecturers' observations on aspects of nurse prescribing training. Nurse Education Today 26(7), 538–544.

Bradley E. & Nolan P. (2007). Impact of nurse prescribing: a qualitative study. Journal of Advanced Nursing 59, 120–128.

Brandon D. (1991). Innovation Without Change: Consumer Power in Psychiatric Services. Macmillan Education.

Brimblecombe N. (2005) The changing relationship between mental health nurses and psychiatrists in the United Kingdom. Journal of Advanced Nursing 49(4), 344–353.

Brimblecombe N., Tingle A., Tumore R. et al. (2007). Implementing holistic practices in mental health nursing: a national consultation. International Journal of Nursing Studies 44(3), 339–348.

BNF (2008). BNF Edition 55. British Medical Association, London. Accessed at: http://www.bnf.org.uk

Brooten D., Naylor M.D. & York R. (2002). Lessons learned from testing the quality cost model of advanced practice nursing (APN) transitional care. Journal of Nursing Scholarship 34(4), 369–375.

Brooks N., Otway C., Rashid C., et al. (2001). The patient's view: the benefits and limitations of nurse prescribing. British Journal of Community Nursing 6, 342–348.

Brown S. (1997). Excess mortality of schizophrenia. A meta-analysis. British Journal of Psychiatry 171, 502–508.

Brown S., Inskip H. & Barraclough B. (2000). Causes of excess mortality of schizophrenia. British Journal of Psychiatry 177, 212–217

Bruce M.S. (1990). The anxiogenic effects of caffeine. Postgraduate Medical Journal 66, S18–S24.

Brugha T.S., Bebbington P.E. & Jenkins R. (1999a). A difference that matters: comparisons of structured and semi-structured psychiatric diagnostic interviews in the general population. Psychological Medicine 29(5), 1013–1020.

Brugha T.S., Nienhuis F.J., Bagchi D., Smith J. & Meltzer H. (1999b). The survey form of SCAN: the feasibility of using experienced lay survey interviewers to administer a semi-structured systematic clinical assessment of psychotic and non-psychotic disorders. Psychological Medicine 29, 703–711.

Bryne M.K., Deane F.P. & Coombs T. (2005). Nurse's beliefs and knowledge about medications are associated with their difficulties using patient treatment adherence strategies. Journal of Mental Health 14, 513–521.

Buchan J. & Calman (2005). Skill mix and policy changes in the health workforce: nurses in advanced roles. OECD Health Working Papers No. 17. OECD Publishing, Paris.

Burns T. & Lloyd H. (2004). Is a team approach based on staff meetings cost effective in the delivery of mental health care? Current Opinion in Psychiatry 17(4), 311–314.

Burris K.D., Molski T.F., Xu C., et al. (2002). Aripiprazole, a novel antipsychotic, is a high-affinity partial agonist at human dopamine D2 receptors. The Journal of Pharmacology and Experimental Therapeutics 302, 381–389.

Bushe S. & Leonard B. (2004). Association between atypical antipsychotic agents and type 2 diabetes: review of prospective clinical data. British Journal of Psychiatry Supplement 47, S87–S93

Campbell C.D., Musil C.M. & Zausziewski J.A. (1998). Practice patterns of advanced practice psychiatric nurses. Journal of American Psychiatric Nurses Association 4(4), 111–120.

Carr N., Bayliss J. & Nolan P. (2002). Report of an Educational Visit to the USA. Perceptions on Nurse Prescribing. South Staffordshire NHS Trust.

Carrillo J.A., Herraiz A.G., Ramos S.I., et al. (1998). Effects of caffeine withdrawal from the diet on the metabolism of clozapine in schizophrenic patients. Journal of Clinical Psychopharmacology 18, 311–316.

Carrillo J.A., Herraiz A.G., Ramos S.I., et al. (2003). Role of the smoking-induced cytochrome P450 (CYP)1A2 and polymorphic CYP2D6 in steady state concentration of olanzapine. Journal of Clinical Psychopharmacology 23, 119–127.

Carroll K.M., Ball S.A. & Martino S. (2008). Computer-assisted delivery of cognitive behavioural therapy for addiction: a randomised trial of CBT4CBT. American Journal of Psychiatry 165, 881–888.

Chadwick P., Birchwood M. & Trower P. (1996). Cognitive therapy for delusions, voices and paranoia. John Wiley & Sons, Chichester.

Chaplin R. & Kent A. (1998). Informing patients about tardive dyskinesia. British Journal of Psychiatry 172, 78–81.

Chrzanowski W.K., Marcus R.N., Torbeyns A., et al. (2006). Effectiveness of long-term aripiprazole therapy in patients with acutely relapsing or chronic, stable schizophrenia: a 52-week, open-label comparison with olanzapine. Psychopharmacology 189, 259–266.

Coffey M. & Jenkins E. (2002). Power and control: forensic community mental health nurses' perceptions of team working, legal sanction and compliance. Journal of Psychiatric and Mental Health Nursing 9, 521–529.

College of Nurses of Ontario (2005a). Legislation and Regulation. RHPA: Scope of Practice, Controlled Acts Model. Reference document. College of Nurses of Ontario, Toronto.

College of Nurses of Ontario (2005b). Practice Standard: Medication. College of Nurses of Ontario, Toronto.

Connolly M. & Kelly C. (2005). Lifestyle and physical health in schizophrenia. Advances in Psychiatric Treatment 11, 125–132.

Cookson J., Taylor D. & Katona C. (2002). Use of Drugs in Psychiatry. Gaskell, London.

Cooney J.L., Cooney N.L., Pilkey D.T., et al. (2003). Effects of nicotine deprivation on urges to drink and smoke in alcoholic smokers. Addiction 98, 913–921.

Cooper J.E. (1994). ICD-10 Classification of Mental and Behavioural Disorders. Churchill Livingstone, Edinburgh.

Cooper N., Blackwell D., Taylor G., et al. (2000) Pharmacists' perceptions of nurse prescribing of emergency contraception. British Journal of Community Nursing 5(3), 126–131.

Cott C. (1998). Structure and meaning in multidisciplinary teamwork. Sociology of Health and Illness 20, 848–873.

Courtenay M. & Carey N. (2007). A review of the impact and effectiveness of nurse-led care in dermatology. Journal of Clinical Nursing 16(1), 122–128.

Courtenay M. & Carey N. (2008). Nurse independent prescribing and nurse supplementary prescribing practice: national survey. Journal of Advanced Nursing 61(3), 291–299.

Courtenay M., Carey N., James J., et al. (2007). An evaluation of a specialist nurse prescriber on diabetes in-patient service delivery. Practical Diabetes International 24, 1–6.

Craddock N., Antebi A., Attenburrow M.-J., et al. (2008). Wake-up call for British psychiatry. British Journal of Psychiatry 193, 6–9.

Cramer J. & Rosenheck R. (1999). Enhancing medication compliance for people with serious mental illness. Journal of Nervous and Mental Disease 187(1), 53–55.

Crisp A.H., Gelder M., Goddard E., et al. (2005). Stigmatization of people with mental illness: a follow-up study within the changing minds campaign of the Royal College of Psychiatrists. World Psychiatry 4, 106–134.

CSIP-NIMHE (2006). Our choices in mental health: a framework for improving choice for people who use mental health services and their carers. CSIP-NIMHE, London.

Curtis L. & Netten A. (2007). The costs of training a nurse practitioner in primary care: the importance of allowing the cost of education and training when making decisions about changing the professional-mix. Journal of Nursing Management 15, 449–457.

Daumit G.L., Goldberg R.W., Anthony C., et al. (2005). Physical activity patterns in adults with severe mental illness. Journal of Nervous and Mental Disease 193, 641–646.

Davies C. (2000). Getting health professionals to work together. British Medical Journal 320, 1021–1022.

Dawson P.J. (1997). Is there anyone there? Psychiatric nursing meets biological psychiatry. Nursing Inquiry 4, 167–172.

Day J.C., Bentall R.P., Roberts C., et al. (2005a). Attitudes toward antipsychotic medication: the impact of clinical variables and relationships with health professionals. Archives of General Psychiatry 62, 717–724.

Day J.C., Wood G., Dewey M., et al. (1995b). A self-rating scale for measuring neuroleptic side effects. Validation in a group of schizophrenic patients. British Journal of Psychiatry 166, 650–653.

Dean B., Schachter M., Vincent C. et al. (2002). Causes of prescribing errors in hospital inpatients: a prospective study. The Lancet 359(315), 1373–1378.

Dementia UK (2007). Dementia UK. Project report. Alzheimer's Society, London.

Department of Health and Social Security (1986). Neighbourhood nursing: A focus for care. Report of the community nursing review (Cumberlege report). HMSO, London.

Dickerson F., Pater A. & Origoni A. (2002). Health behaviours and health status of older women with schizophrenia. Psychiatric Services 53(7), 882–884.

Disability Rights Commission (2006). Equal treatment: closing the gap. DRC. Accessed at: http://www.equalityhumanrights.com/Documents/Formal_investigations/HEALTH4.pdf.

DoH (1989). Report of the Advisory Group on Nurse Prescribing (Crown report). Department of Health, London.

DoH (1996a). The patients charter and you, a charter for England. HMSO, London.

DoH (1996b). Report of an independent survey of drug treatment services in England. The task force to review services for drug misusers. HMSO, London.

DoH (1999a). Review of prescribing, supply and administration of medicines. Final report. Department of Health, London.

DoH (1999b). Making a difference. HMSO, London.

DoH (1999c). A national service framework for mental health. Modern standards and service models. Stationary Office, London.

DoH (2000). The NHS plan. HMSO, London.

DoH (2001). The Journey to recovery – The government's vision for mental health care. HMSO, London.

DoH (2002). Mental health policy implementation guide: dual diagnosis good practice guide. Department of Health, London.

DoH (2003). Supplementary prescribing by nurses and pharmacists within the NHS in England. HMSO, London.

DoH (2004a). Achieving timely 'simple' discharge from hospital. HMSO, London.

DoH (2004b). Building a safer NHS for patients: improving medication safety. Department of Health, London.

DoH (2005a). Supporting people with long-term conditions. An NHS and social care model to support local innovation and integration. Department of Health, London.

DoH (2005b). New ways of working for psychiatrists. Final report 'But not the end of the story'. Department of Health, London.

DoH (2006a). Medicines matters: A guide to mechanisms for the prescribing, supply and administration of medicines. Department of Health, London.

DoH (2006b). Improving patients' access to medicines: a guide to implementing nurse and pharmacist independent prescribing within the NHS in England. Department of Health, London.

DoH (2006c). From values to action: the chief nursing officers review of mental health nursing. Department of Health, London.

DoH (2006d). Choosing health: supporting the physical health needs of people with serious mental illness. Department of Health, London.

DoH (2006e). Modernising nursing careers. National Assembly for Wales, Cardiff.

DoH (2007a). New ways of working for everyone – best practice toolkit. Department of Health, London.

DoH (2007b). Creating capable teams approach (CCTA). Best practice guidance to support the implementation of new ways of working and new roles. Department of Health, London.

DoH (2007c). Safe. Sensible. Social. The next steps in the National Alcohol Strategy. Department of Health, London.

DoH (2007d). A recipe for care – not a single ingredient. Department of Health, London.

DoH (2008a). Medicines management: everybody's business. Department of Health, London.

DoH (2008b). Mental Health Act 2007. Accessed at: http://www.dh.gov.uk/en/Healthcare/NationalServiceFrameworks/Mentalhealth/DH_078743

DoH (2008c). A high-quality workforce. NHS next stage review. Department of Health, London.

DoH (2008d). Supporting successful nurse prescribing. Department of Health, London.

DoH/CSIP (2007). Guidance statement on fidelity and best practice for crisis services. Department of Health, London.

Duncan L., Heathcote J., Djurdjev O. et al. (2001). Screening for renal disease using serum creatine: who are we missing? Nephrol Dial Transplant 16, 1042–1046.

El-Zayadi A.R. (2006). Heavy smoking and liver. World Journal of Gastroenterology 12, 6098–6101.

Farmer A., Korszun A. & Owen M.J. (2008). Medical disorders in people with recurrent depression. British Journal of Psychiatry 192, 351–355.

Fawcett B. & Karban K. (2005). Contemporary Mental Health: Theory, Policy and Practice. Routledge, London.

Felton A. & Stickey T. (2004). Pedagogy, power and service user involvement. Journal of Psychiatric and Mental Health Nursing 11, 89–98.

First M.B., Gibbon M., Spitzer R.L. et al. (1997). Structured Clinical Interview for DSM-IV Axis II Personality Disorder (SCID-II). American Psychiatric Press, Washington, DC.

Fisher S.E. & Vaughan-Cole B. (2003). Similarities and differences in clients treated and in medications prescribed by APRNs and psychiatrists in a CMHC. Archives of Psychiatric Nursing XVII(3), 101–107.

Fisher R. (2005). Relationships in nurse prescribing in district nursing practice in England: a preliminary investigation. International Journal of Nursing Practice 11(3), 102–107.

Fitzpatrick R. (1991). Surveys of patient satisfaction: 1 – Important general considerations. British Medical Journal 302(6781), 887–889.

Folstein M.F., Folstein S.E. & McHugh H.R. (1975). Mini-mental state: a practical method for grading the cognitive state of patients for the clinician. Journal of Psychiatric Research 12, 189–198.

Food Health Forum (2008). The links between diet and behaviour: the influence of nutrition on mental health. Report of an inquiry held by the Associate Parliamentary Food and Health Forum, HMSO.

Food Standards Agency (2004). Survey of caffeine levels in hot beverages. FSA. Accessed at: http://www.food.gov.uk.

Foucault M. (1974). The Order of Things. Tavistock, London.

Frances A., Pincus H.A. & First M.B. (1994). Diagnostic and Statistical Manual of Mental Disorder-IV. American Psychiatric Association, Washington.

Fredholm B.B., Battig K., Holmen J., et al. (1999). Actions of coffee in the brain with special reference to factors that contribute to its widespread use. Pharmacological Reviews 51(1), 83–133.

Freeman A.J., Dore G.J., Law M.G., et al. (2001). Estimating progression in cirrhosis in chronic hepatitis C. Hepatology 34, 809–816.

Gallagher J., Ruskin A. & O'Gara C. (2006). Nurse prescribing in addiction services: client benefits. Nursing Standard 20, 42–44.

Garcia-Unzueta M.T., Herran A., Sierra-Biddle D., et al. (2003). Alterations of liver function tests in patients treated with antipsychotics. Journal of Clinical Laboratory Analysis 17, 216–218.

Garland M.R., Hallahan B., McNamara M., et al. (2007). Lipids and essential fatty acids in patients presenting with self-harm. British Journal of Psychiatry 190, 112–117.

Gask L. (2005). Role of specialists in common chronic diseases. British Medical Journal 330, 651–653.

Gee M. (2007). New ways of working threatens the future of the psychiatric profession. Psychiatric Bulletin 31, 315.

Gelder M., Mayou R. & Cowen P. (2004). Shorter Oxford Textbook of Psychiatry, Part 2. Oxford University Press, Oxford.

Gilmore I. & Sheron N. (2007). Reducing the harm of alcohol in the UK. British Medical Journal 335, 1271–1272.

Goldberg D. & Huxley P. (1992). Common Mental Disorders. Routledge, London.

Gooden J.M. & Jackson E. (2004). Attitudes of registered nurses towards nurse practitioners. Journal of the American Academy of Nurse Practitioners 16, 360–364.

Gossop M. & Moos R. (2008). Substance misuse among older adults: a neglected but treated problem. Addiction 103, 347–348.

Gough S.C.L. & O'Donovan M.C. (2005). Clustering of metabolic comorbidity in schizophrenia: a genetic contribution. Journal of Psychopharmacology 19, 47–55.

Gournay K. (1995). What to do with nursing models. Journal of Psychiatric and Mental Health Nursing 2, 325–327.

Granby T. (2007). Are you receiving appropriate support. Accessed at: http://www.npc.co.uk/presentations/trudy_afternoon.ppt

Grant G., Page D. & Maybury C. (2007). Introducing nurse prescribing in a memory clinic: staff experiences. Mental Health Nursing 27, 9–13.

Grantham G., McMillan V., Dunn S., et al. (2006). Patient self-medication – a change in hospital practice. Journal of Clinical Nursing 15(8), 962–970.

Gravel K., Legare F. & Graham I.D. (2006). Barriers and facilitators to implementing shared decision making in clinical practice: a systematic review of health professionals' perceptions. Implementation Science 1, 1–15.

Gray R., Leese M. & Bindman J. (2006). Adherence therapy for people with schizophrenia. British Journal of Psychiatry 189, 508–514.

Gray R., Parr A. & Robson D. (2005a). Has tardive dyskinesia disappeared? Mental Health Practice 8, 20–22.

Gray R., Parr A.-M. & Brimblecombe N. (2005b). Mental health nurse supplementary prescribing: mapping process 1 year after implementation. Psychiatric Bulletin 29, 295–297.

Gray R., Rofail D., Allen J., et al. (2005c). A survey of patient satisfaction with and subjective experience of treatment with antipsychotic medication. Journal of Advanced Nursing 52, 31–37.

Gray R., Wykes T. & Edmonds M. (2004). Effect of a medication management training package for nurses on clinical outcomes for patients with schizophrenia. British Journal of Psychiatry 185, 157–162.

Gray R., Wykes T. & Gournay K. (2002). From compliance to concordance: a review of the literature on interventions to enhance compliance with antipsychotic medication. Journal of Psychiatric and Mental Health Nursing 9, 227–284.

Greenberg G.A., Myer J., Sernyak M., et al. (2006). Access of behavioural health patients to prescribing professionals. General Hospital Psychiatry 28, 249–254.

Greenwood N., Key A., Burns T., et al. (1999). Satisfaction with inpatient psychiatric services: relationship to patient and treatment factors. British Journal of Psychiatry 174, 159–163.

Griffiths S.R. (1988). Community care: agenda for action. HMSO, London.

Guillaume L., Cooper R., Avery A., et al. (2008). Supplementary prescribing by community and primary care pharmacists: an analysis of PACT data, 2004–2006. Journal of Clinical Pharmacy and Therapeutics 33, 11–16.

Haddock G., Barrowclough C., Tarrier N., et al. (2003). Cognitive behavioural therapy and motivational intervention for schizophrenia and substance misuse. British Journal of Psychiatry 183, 418–426.

Haddock G. (1994). Delusion Rating Scale. www.mentalhealthnurse.co.uk/images/Assessment%20Tools

Hall J., Cantrill J. & Noyce P. (2006). Why don't trained community nurse prescribers prescribe? Journal of Clinical Nursing 15(4), 403–412.

Hamann J., Langer B., Busch R et al. (2004) Medical decision making in antipsychotic drug choice. American Journal of Psychiatry 161, 1301–1304.

Hamblet C. (2000). Obstacles to defining the role of the nurse. Nursing Standard 14, 34–37.

Hamilton B., Manias E., Maude P., et al. (2004). Perspectives of a nurse, a social worker and a psychiatrist regarding patient assessment in acute inpatient psychiatry settings: a case study approach. Journal of Psychiatric and Mental Health Nursing 11, 683–689.

Happell B., Pinikahana J. & Roper C. (2002). Attitudes of postgraduate nursing students towards consumer participation in mental health services and the role of the consumer academic. International Journal of Mental Health Nursing 11, 240–250.

Harborne G. & Jones A. (2008). Supplementary prescribing: a new way of working for psychiatrists and nurses. Psychiatric Bulletin 32, 136–139.

Harniman B. (2007). Personal reflections on non-medical prescribing in substance misuse. Nurse Prescribing 5, 211–213.

Harris N., Lovell K. & Day J.C. (2007). Mental health practitioner's attitude towards maintenance neuroleptic treatment for people with schizophrenia. Journal of Psychiatric and Mental Health Nursing 14(2), 113–119.

Harrison A. (2003). Mental health service users' views of nurse prescribing. Nurse Prescribing 1, 78–85.

Havard A., Teeson M., Darke S., et al. (2006). Depression among heroin users: 12-month outcomes from the Australian treatment outcome study (ATOS). Journal of Substance Abuse Treatment 30, 355–362.

Hay A., Bradley E. & Nolan P. (2004). Supplementary nurse prescribing. Nursing Standard 18(41), 33–9.

Haynes R.B., McKibbon K.A., Kanani R. (1996) Systematic review of randomised trials of interventions to assist patients to follow prescriptions for medications. Lancet 348(9024), 383–386.

Healthcare Commission (2006). Acute hospital portfolio reviews 2005–2006. Guide to medicines management in trusts providing mental health services. Accessed at: http://www.healthcarecommission.org.uk

Healthcare Commission (2007a). Acute inpatient mental health service review. Accessed at: http://www.healthcarecommission.org.uk

Healthcare Commission (2007b). Talking about medicines: the management of medicines in trusts providing mental health services. Commission for Healthcare Audit and Inspection, London. Accessed at: http://www.healthcarecommission.org.uk

Healy D. (2005). Psychiatric Drugs Explained. Elsevier, Edinburgh.

Helgason L. (1990) Twenty years' follow-up of first psychiatric presentation for schizophrenia: what could have been prevented? Acta Psychiatrica Scandinavica 81(3), 231–235.

Hemingway S. (2004). The mental health nurse's perspective on implementing nurse prescribing. Nurse Prescribing 2(1), 37–44.

Hemingway S. & Davies J. (2005). Non-medical prescribing education: how do we meet the needs of the diverse nursing specialisms? Nurse Prescriber 2, e58, doi:10.1017/S1467115805000581.

Hennekens C., Hennekens A., Hollar D., et al. (2005). Schizophrenia and increased risks of cardiovascular disease. American Heart Journal 150(6), 1115–1121.

Himelhoch S., Lehman A., Kreyenbuhl J., et al. (2004). Prevalence of chronic obstructive pulmonary disease among those with serious mental illness. American Journal Psychiatry 161, 2317–2319.

Hobson R.J. & Sewell G.J. (2006). Risks and concerns about supplementary prescribing: survey of primary and secondary care pharmacists. Pharmacy World & Science 28, 76–90.

Holt R.I. (2005). Obesity – an epidemic of the twenty-first century: an update for psychiatrists. Journal of Psychopharmacology 19(6), 6–15.

Home Office (2001). The misuse of Drugs Regulations 2001. Statutory Instrument 2001, No. 3998. Accessed at: http://www.opsi.gov.uk/si/si2001/20013998.htm

Horrocks S., Anderson E. & Salisbury C. (2002). Systematic review of whether nurse practitioners working in primary care can provide equivalent care to doctors. British Medical Journal 324, 819–823.

Horton R. (2002). Nurse-prescribing in the UK: right but also wrong. Lancet 359, 1875.

Howard P.B. & Greiner D. (1997). Constraints to advanced psychiatric-mental health nursing practice. Archives of Psychiatric Nursing 11(4), 198–209.

Institute of Medicine (1995). Weighing the Options: Criteria for Evaluating Eight Management Programmes. National Academy Press, Washington.

ICN (2004). Implementing Nurse Prescribing: An Updated Review of Current Practice Internationally. ICN, Geneva.

Jacobs J.T. (2005). Treatment of depressive disorders in split versus integrated therapy and comparisons of prescriptive practices of psychiatrists and advanced practice registered nurses. Archives of Psychiatric Nursing 12, 256–63

Jack B. & Merriman A. (2008). Dying without pain: nurses giving morphine in Uganda. European Journal of Palliative Care 15, 92–95.

Jagwe J. & Merriman A. (2007). Uganda: delivering analgesia in rural Africa: opioid availability and nurse prescribing. Journal of Pain and Symptom Management 33, 547–551.

Joint British Society (2005). JBS 2: Joint British Societies' guidelines on prevention of cardiovascular disease in clinical practice. Heart 91, 1–52.

Jones A. (2006a). Acute psychiatric inpatient wards. Nurse Prescriber e0, 1-5, doi: 10.1017/S1467115806000010.

Jones A. (2006b). Multidisciplinary team working: collaboration and conflict. International Journal of Mental Health Nursing 15, 19–28.

Jones A. (2006c). Supplementary prescribing: relationships between nurses and psychiatrists on hospital psychiatric wards. Journal of Psychiatric and Mental Health Nursing 13, 3–11.

Jones A. (2006d). Supplementary prescribing: potential ways to reform hospital psychiatric care. Journal of Psychiatric and Mental Health Nursing 13, 132–138.

Jones A. (2006e). Born in the USA. Mental Health Practice 9(6), 44.

Jones M. (2007). Psychopharmacology for nurse prescribers. Nurse Prescribing Conference Report. Surrey and Borders NHS Trust (Unpublished report).

Jones A. (2008). Exploring independent nurse prescribing for mental health settings. Journal of Psychiatric and Mental Health Nursing 15, 109–117.

Jones A., Doyle V., Pyke S., et al. (2005). New roles for nurses and psychiatrists in the management of long-term conditions. Mental Health Practice 9(3), 16–20.

Jones A. & Harborne G. (2005). Supplementary prescribing in hospital settings. Mental Health Practice 9, 38–40.

Jones A. & Jones M. (2005). Mental health nurse prescribing: issues for the UK. Journal of Psychiatric and Mental Health Nursing 12, 527–535.

Jones A. & Jones M. (2008a). Helping people on acute wards to stop smoking. Mental Health Practice 11, 18–21.

Jones C., Cormac I., Silveira da Mota Neto J.I., et al. (2004). Cognitive behaviour therapy for schizophrenia. The Cochrane Database of Systematic Reviews, Issue 4. Art No.: CD000524.1 0.1002/14651858.CD000524.pud2.

Jones M. (2004). Nurse prescribing: a case study in policy influence. Journal of Nursing Management 12, 266–272.

Jones M., Bennett J., Lucas B., et al. (2007). Mental health nurse prescribing: experiences of mental health nurses, psychiatrists and patients. Journal of Advanced Nursing 58(6), 1–9.

Jones M. & Jones A. (2006). Prescribing new ways of working. Mental Health Practice 9(6), 20–22.

Jones M. & Jones A. (2007a). Choice as an intervention to promote well-being: the role of the nurse prescriber. Journal of Psychiatric and Mental Health Nursing 15, 75–81.

Jones M. & Jones A. (2007b). Delivering the choice agenda as a framework to manage adverse effects: a mental health nurse perspective on prescribing psychiatric medication. Journal of Psychiatric and Mental Health Nursing 14, 418–423.

Jones M. & Jones A. (2008b). Promotion of choice in the care of people with bipolar disorder: a mental health nursing perspective. Journal of Psychiatric and Mental Health Nursing 15, 87–92.

Jordan S., Tunnicliffe C. & Sykes A. (2002). Minimizing side effects: the clinical impact of nurse-administered 'side effect' checklist. Journal of Advanced Nursing 37(2), 155–165.

Jordan S., Knight J. & Pointon D. (2004). Monitoring adverse drug reactions: scales, profiles, and checklists. International Nursing Review 51, 208–221.

Kaas M.J., Dahl D., Dehn D., et al. (1998). Barriers to prescriptive practice for psychiatric/mental health clinical nurse specialists. Clinical Nurse Specialist 12(5), 200–204.

Kaas M.J., Dehn D., Dahl D., et al. (2000). A view of prescriptive practice collaboration: perspectives of psychiatric mental health clinical nurse specialists and psychiatrists. Archives of Psychiatric Nursing XIV(5), 222–234.

Kaas M.J. & Markley J.M. (1998). A national perspective on prescriptive authority for advanced practice psychiatric nurses. Journal of American Psychiatric Nurses Association 4(6), 190–198.

Kaplan L. & Brown M.A. (2007). The transition of nurse practitioners to changes in prescriptive authority. Journal of Nursing Scholarship 39, 184–190.

Katon W., von Korff M., Lin E., et al. (2001). Rethinking practitioner roles in chronic illness: the specialist, primary care physician, and the practice nurse. General Hospital Psychiatry 23, 138–144.

Kavanagh D.J., Greenaway L., Jenner L., et al. (2000). Contrasting views and experience of health professionals on the management of comorbid substance misuse and mental disorders. Australian and New Zealand Journal of Psychiatry 34, 279–289.

Kemp R., Hayward P. & Applewhaite G. (1996). Compliance therapy in psychotic patients: randomised controlled trial. British Medical Journal 312, 345–349.

King R.L. (2004). Nurses' perceptions of their pharmacology educational needs. Journal of Advanced Nursing 45(4), 392–400.

Koenig H.G. & Blazer D.G. (1992). Epidemiology of geriatric affective disorders. Clinical Geriatric Medicine 8, 235–251.

Koplan K.E., David S.P. & Rigotti N.A. (2008). Smoking cessation. British Medical Journal 336, 217.

Lam D.H. & Wong G. (1997). Prodromes, coping strategies, insight and social functioning in biopolar affective disorder. Psychological Medicine 27, 1091–1100.

Lammers J. & Happell B. (2004). Mental health reforms and their impact on consumer and carer participation: a perspective from Victoria. Issues in Mental Health Nursing 25, 261–276.

Lanceley A., Savage J., Menon U., et al. (2008). Influences on multidisciplinary team decision making. International Journal of Gynaecological Cancer 18(2), 215–222.

Latter S. (2005). Promoting concordance in prescribing interactions: the evidence base and implications for the new generation of prescribers. In: M. Courtney & M. Griffiths (Eds.). Independent and Supplementary Prescribing: An Essential Guide. University Press, Cambridge.

Latter S. & Courtenay M. (2004). Effectiveness of nurse prescribing: a review of the literature. Journal of Clinical Nursing 13, 26–32.

Latter S., Maben J., Myall M., et al. (2005). An Evaluation of Extended Formulary Independent Nurse Prescribing. University of Southampton, Southampton.

Latter S., Maben J., Myall M., et al. (2007). Evaluating prescribing competencies and standards used in nurse independent prescribers' prescribing consultations. Journal of Research in Nursing 12, 7–26.

Laungani P. (2002). Mindless psychiatry and dubious ethics. Counselling Psychiatry Quarterly 15, 23–33.

Laurant M.G.H., Hermens R.P.M.G., Braspenning C.C., et al. (2004). Impact of nurse practitioners on workload of general practitioners: randomised controlled trial. British Medical Journal 328, 927.

Lawrence R., Bradshaw T. & Mairs H. (2006). Group cognitive behavioural therapy for schizophrenia: a systematic review of the literature. Journal of Psychiatric and Mental Health Nursing 13, 673–681.

Layard R. (2006). The depression report: a new deal for depression and anxiety disorders. Centre for Economic Performance, London School of Economics, London.

Lazaro F., Kulinskaya E. & Tobiansky R. (2001). Crisis intervention: the professionals' perspective. Psychiatric Bulletin 25, 95–98.

Leape L.L., Bates D.W., Cullen D.J. et al. (1995). Systems analysis of adverse drug events. ADE prevention study group. Journal of the American Medical Association 274(1), 35–43.

Leathard H.L. (2001). Understanding medicines: conceptual analysis of nurses needs for knowledge and understanding of pharmacology. Nurse Education Today 21, 260–271.

Lecompte D. & Pelc I. (1996). A cognitive-behavioural program to improve compliance with medication in patients with schizophrenia. International Journal of Mental Health 25(1), 51–56.

Lenton S. & Single E. (1998). The definition of harm reduction. Drugs and Alcohol Review 17, 213–220.

Leppard J. (2008). Running a clozapine clinic: considerations and challenges. Nurse Prescribing 6, 162–167.

Lewis-Evans A. & Jester A. (2004). Nurse prescribers' experiences of prescribing. Journal of Clinical Nursing 13, 796–805.

Lieberman J.A., Stroup T.S., McEvoy J.P., et al. (2005). Effectiveness of antipsychotic drugs in patients with chronic schizophrenia. New England Journal of Medicine 353, 1209–1223.

Lim A.G., Honey M. & Kilpatrick J. (2007). Framework for teaching pharmacology to prepare graduate nurse for prescribing in New Zealand. Nurse Education Practice 7, 348–353.

Lim W.S., Gammack J.K., Niekerk J.K., et al. (2006). Omega-3 fatty acid for the prevention of dementia. Cochrane Database of Systematic Reviews 2006, Issue 1. Art No.: CD005379, doi: 10.1002/14651858.CD005379.pub2.

Lingjaerde O., Ahlfors U.G., Bech S.J. et al. (1987). The UKU side effect rating scale: A new comprehensive rating scale for psychotropic drugs and a cross-sectional study of side effects in neuroleptic-treated patients. Acta Psychiatrica Scandinavica 76, s334, 1–100.

Lockwood E.B. & Fealy G.M. (2008). Journal of Nursing Management Nurse prescribing as an aspect of future role expansion: the views of Irish clinical nurse specialists 16(7), 813–820.

Loh A., Leonhart R., Wills C.E., et al. (2007). The impact of patient participation on adherence and clinical outcome in primary care of depression. Patient Education and Counselling 65, 69–75.

Loh A., Simon D. & Hennig K. (2006). The assessment of depressive patients' involvement in decision making in audio taped primary care consultations. Patient Education and Counselling 63, 314–318.

Lupton D. (1997). Consumerism, reflexivity and the medical encounter. Social Science and Medicine 45(3), 373–381.

Luker K.A., Austin L., Willock J. et al. (1997). Nurses' and GP's views of the nurse prescribers' formulary. Nursing Standard 11(22), 33–38.

Luker K.A., Austin L., Hogg C., et al. (1998). Nurse-patient relationships: the context of nurse prescribing. Journal of Advanced Nursing 28, 235–242.

MacManus E. & Fitzpatrick C. (2007). Alcohol dependence and mood state in a population receiving methadone maintenance treatment. Irish Journal of Psychological Medicine 24, 19–22.

Makoul G., Arntson P. & Schofield T. (2005). Health promotion in primary care: physician-patient communication and decision making about prescription medications. Social Science and Medicine 41(99), 1241–1254.

Malone D., Fineberg A.N. & Gale T.M. (2004). What is the usual length of stay in a psychiatric ward. International Journal of Psychiatry in Clinical Practice 8, 53–56.

Malone D., Marriott S., Newton-Howes G., et al. (2007). Community mental health teams (CMHTs) for people with severe mental illnesses and disordered personality. Cochrane Database of Systematic Reviews 2007, Issue 2. Art. No.: CD000270, doi:10.1002/14651858.CD000270.pub2.

Mason T., Carlisle C., Watkins C., et al. (2001). Stigma and social exclusion. Routledge, London.

McCann T. & Hemingway S. (2003). Models of prescriptive authority for mental health nurse practitioners. Journal of Psychiatric and Mental Health Nursing 10, 743–749.

McCann T.V. & Baker H. (2002). Community mental health nurses and authority to prescribe medications: the way forward. Journal of Psychiatric and Mental Health Nursing 9, 175–182.

McCann T.V., Baird J. & Lu S. (2008). Mental health professionals' attitude towards consumer participation in inpatient units. Journal of Psychiatric and Mental Health Nursing 15, 10–16.

McCann T.V. & Clark E. (2008). Attitudes of patients towards mental health nurse prescribing of antipsychotic agents. International Journal of Nursing Practice 14, 115–121.

McCreadie R.G. (2003). Diet, smoking and cardiovascular risk in people with schizophrenia. British Journal of Psychiatry 183, 534–539.

McCreadie R.G., Kelly C., Connolly M.A., et al. (2005). Dietary improvements in people with schizophrenia. British Journal of Psychiatry 187, 346–351.

McCreadie R.G., Macdonald E., Blacklock C., et al. (1998). Dietary intake of schizophrenic patients in Nithsdale, Scotland: case-control study. British Medical Journal 317, 784–785.

McEvoy J.P., Apperson L.J., Applebaum P.S., et al. (1989). Insight in schizophrenia: its relationship to acute psychopathology. Journal of Nervous Mental Disorder 177, 43–47.

McGorry P.D. (2000). The scope for preventative strategies in early psychosis: logic, evidence and momentum. In: M. Birchwood, D. Fowler & C. Jackson (Eds.). Early Intervention in Psychosis: A Guide to Concepts, Evidence and Interventions, pp. 3–27. Wiley, Chichester.

McGraw C. & Drennan V. (2001). Self administration of medicine and older people. Nursing Standard 15(18), 33–36.

McIver S. (1999). Public involvement in primary care: implications for primary care groups. Nursing Times Research 4(4), 245–256.

McKinley R.K. & Middleton J.F. (1999). What do patients want from doctors? Content analysis of written patient agendas for the consultation. British Journal of General Practice 49, 796–800.

Meaney A.M. & O'Keane V. (2002). Prolactin and schizophrenia. Clinical consequences of hyperprolactinaemia. Life Sciences 71, 979–992.

Meier P.S., Barrowclough C. & Donmall M.C. (2005). The role of the therapeutic alliance in the treatment of substance misuse: a critical review of the literature. Addiction 100, 304–316.

Melia K.M. (1987). Learning and working: the occupational socialisation of nurses. Tavistock, London.

Meltzer H.Y. & Okayli G. (1995). Reduction of suicidality during clozapine treatment of neuroleptic-resistant schizophrenia: impact on risk-benefit assessment. American Journal of Psychiatry 152(2), 183–190.

Menezes P.O., Johnson S., Thornicroft G., et al. (1996). Drug and alcohol problems among individuals with severe mental illness in South London. British Journal of Psychiatry 168, 612–619.

Meyer J.C., Summers R.S. & Moller H. (2001). Randomised, controlled trial of prescribing training in a South African province. Medical Education 35, 833–840.

Miles K., Seitio O. & McGilvray M. (2006). Nurse prescribing in low-resource settings: professional considerations. International Nursing Review 53, 290–296.

Miller W.R. & Rollnick S. (2004). Talking oneself into change: motivational interviewing, stages of change, and therapeutic process. Journal of Cognitive Psychotherapy 18, 299–308.

Moncrieff J. (1997). Psychiatric imperialism: the medicalisation of modern living [reprinted from Soundings, Issue 6, Summer]. Lawrence and Wishart, London.

Moos R., Brennan P., Schutte K., et al. (2004). High-risk alcohol consumption and late-life alcohol use problems. American Journal of Public Health 94, 1985–1991.

Moussavi S., Chatterji S., Verdes E., et al. (2007). Depression, chronic diseases, and decrements in health: results from the world health surveys. Lancet 370, 851–858.

Munro A., Watson H.E. & McFayden A. (2007). Assessing the impact of training on mental health nurses' therapeutic attitudes and knowledge about co-morbidity: a randomised controlled trial. International Journal of Nursing Studies 44, 1430–1438.

Murray A. (2007). Nurse prescribing in older person's mental health. Nurse Prescribing 5, 401–407.

Murray C.J. & Lopez A.D. (1996). Evidence-based health policy – lessons from the global burden of disease study. Science 274, 740–743.

National Audit Office (2006). Prescribing in primary care. Understanding what shapes GPs' prescribing choices and how might these be changed. RAND Corporation, Santa Monica.

National Audit Office (2001). Tackling obesity in England. The Stationary Office, London.

National Collaborating Centre for Mental Health (2004). Self-harm: The short-term physical and psychological management and secondary prevention of self-harm in primary and secondary care. Royal College of Psychiatrists, London.

NHS LA (2008) National Health Service Litigation Authority Report and Accounts2008. Office of Public Sector Information, Surrey.

National Institute of Mental Health in England (NIMHE) (2006). National suicide prevention strategy for England. Annual report on progress 2005. NIMHE, Leeds.

National Nursing and Nursing Education Taskforce (2006a). Myth Busters. Accessed at: http://www.nnet.gov.au/downloads/mythbusters_np.pdf

National Nursing and Nursing Education Taskforce (2006b). National Nurse Prescribing Glossary. Australian Health Ministers' Advisory Council. Accessed at: http://www.nnet.gov.au/downloads/n3et_national_nurse_prescribing_glossary.pdf.

National Obesity Forum (2008). Guidelines on management of adult obesity and overweight in primary care. Accessed at: http://www.nationalobesityforum.org.uk

National Patient Safety Agency (NPSA) (2006). With Safety in Mind: Mental Health Services and Patient Safety. Patient Safety Observatory Report (Mental Health) July 2006. NPSA, London.

National Prescribing Centre (2003). Maintaining competency in prescribing – an outline framework to help nurse supplementary prescribers (update). Accessed at: http://www.npc.nhs.uk

National Prescribing Centre (2004). Patient group directions. A practical guide and framework of competencies for all professionals using patient group directions. Accessed at: www.npc.nhs.uk

National Prescribing Centre (2005a). Improving mental health services by extending the role of nurses in prescribing and supplying medication: good practice guide. NPC, Liverpool.

National Prescribing Centre (2005b). Training non-medical prescribers in practice. NPC, Liverpool.

National Prescribing Centre (2005c). Results of surveying non-medical prescribers. Accessed at: http://www.npc.co.uk/non_medical/Survey_Results_2005.pdf

National Prescribing Centre (2007). A competency framework for shared decision-making with patients: achieving concordance about taking medicines. Accessed at: National Prescribing Centre (2008). Moving towards personalising medicines management: improving outcomes for people through the safe and effective use of medicines. Accessed at: http://www.npc.nhs.uk

National Treatment Agency (2007). Drug misuse and dependence. Guidelines on clinical management. NTA, London.

New Zealand Ministry of Health (1997). Report of the working group advising on the quality and safety issues associated with extending limited prescribing rights to registered nurses: report to the director-general of health. New Zealand Ministry of Health, Wellington.

New Zealand Ministry of Health (1998). Consultation document: nurse prescribing in aged care and child family health. New Zealand Ministry of Health, Wellington.

Ngcongco V.N. & Stark R.D. (1986). The development of a family nurse practitioner programme in Botswana. International Nursing Review 33(1), 9–14.

NICE (2002a). Schizophrenia: core interventions in the treatment and management of schizophrenia in primary and secondary care. Clinical Guideline No. 1, December 2002. NICE, London.

NICE (2002b). Guidance for the use of newer (atypical) antipsychotic drugs for the treatment of schizophrenia. Technology Appraisal Guidance No. 43, June 2002. NICE, London.

NICE (2002c). Nicotine replacement therapy and bupropion for smoking cessation. NICE, London.

NICE (2004a). Guidance on the use of zaleplon, zolpidem and zopiclone for the short-term management of insomnia. Technology Appraisal 77. NICE, London.

NICE (2004b). Eating disorders: core interventions in the treatment and management of anorexia nervosa, bulimia nervosa and related eating disorders. NICE, London.

NICE (2005). The short-term management of disturbed/violent behaviour in psychiatric inpatient settings and emergency departments. NICE, London.

NICE (2006a). Dementia: supporting people with dementia and their carers in health and social care. NICE/SCIE, London.

NICE (2006b). Depression: management of depression in primary and secondary care. Report No. CG23. NICE, London.

NICE (2006c). Bipolar disorder. NICE, London.

NICE (2006d). Smoking cessation. NICE, London.

NICE (2007a). Donepezil, galantamine, rivastigmine, and memantine for Alzheimer's disease. NICE, London.

NICE (2007b). Methadone and buprenorphine for the management of opioid dependence. NICE, London.

NICE (2008). Smoking cessation services in primary care, pharmacies, local authorities and workplaces, particularly for manual working groups, pregnant women and hard to reach communities. NICE, London.

Nilsson M. (1994). Opposition to nurse prescribing in Sweden. Lancet 344, 1077.

Nirodi P. & Mitchell A.J. (2002). The quality of psychotropic drug prescribing in patients in psychiatric units for the elderly. Ageing and Mental Health 6, 191–196.

Noble L.M., Douglas B.C. & Newman S.P. (2001). What do patients expect of psychiatric services? A systematic and critical review of empirical studies. Social Science and Medicine 52(7), 985–998.

Nolan P. (1998). A History of Mental Health Nursing. Nelson Thornes. ISBN 0748737219.

Nolan P. & Bradley E. (2007). The role of the nurse prescriber: the views of mental health and non-mental health nurses. Journal of Psychiatric and Mental Health Nursing 14, 258–266.

Nolan P., Haque M.S., Badger F., et al. (2001). Mental health nurses' perceptions of nurse prescribing. Journal of Advanced Nursing 36, 527–534.

North West Medicines Information Centre (2006). Which medicines need dose adjustment when a patient stops smoking. NWMIC, Liverpool.

Nose M., Barbui C. & Tansella M. (2003). How often do patients with psychosis fail to adhere to treatment programmes? A systematic review. Psychological Medicine 33, 1149–1160.

Nursing & Midwifery Council (2006). Standards of proficiency for nurse and midwife prescribers. NMC, London.

Nursing & Midwifery Council (2007). Standards for medicines management. Accessed at: http://www.nmc-uk.org

Nursing & Midwifery Council (2008). Guidance for Continuing Professional Development for Nurse and Midwife Prescribers. Accessed at: http://www.nmc-uk.org

O'Brien L. & Cole R. (2004). Mental health nursing practice in acute psychiatric close-observation areas. International Journal of Mental Health Nursing 13, 89–99.

O'Donnell C., Donohoe G., Sharkey L. et al. (2003). Compliance therapy: randomised controlled trial in schizophrenia. British Medical Journal 327(7419), 834–836.

O'Keefe C.D., Noordsy D.L., Liss T.B., et al. (2003). Reversal of antipsychotic-associated weight gain. Journal of Clinical Psychiatry 64, 907–912.

O'Shea E. (1999). Factors contributing to medication errors: a literature review. Journal of Clinical Nursing 8, 496–504.

Onyett S. (2002). Teamworking in Mental Health. Palgrave Macmillan, Hampshire.

Onyett S., Heppleston T. & Bushnell D. (1994). A national survey of community mental health teams. Team structure and process. Journal of Mental Health 3, 175–194.

Opie A. (1997). Thinking teams thinking clients: issues of discourse and representation in the work of health care. Sociology of Health & Illness 19, 259–280.

Otway C. (2002). The development needs of nurse prescribers. Nursing Standard 16, 33–38.

Patel M.X., DeZotsa N., Baker D., et al. (2005). Antipsychotic depot medication and attitudes of community psychiatric nurses. Journal of Psychiatric and Mental Health Nursing 12, 237–244.

Patterson M. & Hayes S. (1977). Verbal communication between students in multidisciplinary teams. Medical Education 11, 205–209.

Pekkala E. & Merinder L. (2003). Psychoeducation for Schizophrenia. Cochrane Database of Systematic Reviews, Issue 4. The Cochrane Library, UK.

Perkins D.O., Gu H., Boteva K., et al. (2005). Relationship between duration of untreated psychosis and outcome in first-episode schizophrenia: a critical review and meta-analysis. American Journal of Psychiatry 162, 1785–1804.

Phillips S.J. (2005). A comprehensive look at the legislative issues affecting advanced nursing practice. The Nurse Practitioner 30(1), 14–18.

Poole R. & Bhugra D. (2008). Should psychiatry exist? International Journal of Social Psychiatry 54, 195–196.

Poole R. & Higgo R. (2006). Psychiatric interviewing and assessment. Cambridge University Press, Cambridge.

Porter R. (2002). Madness: A Brief History. Oxford University Press, Oxford.

Public Citizen (2001). Rx R&D Myths: The Case Against the Drug Industry's R&D 'Scare Card'. Public Citizen's Congress Watch, Washington, D.C.

Ramcharan P., Hemingway S. & Flowers K. (2001). A client-centred care for nurse prescribing. Mental Health Nursing 21(5), 6–11.

Ranney L., Melvin C., Lux L., et al. (2006). Systematic review: smoking cessation intervention strategies for adults and adults in special populations. Annals of Internal Medicine 145, 845–856.

Reason J. (1990). Human Error. Cambridge University Press, Cambridge.

Rethink (2006). Stigma and health services. Accessed at: http://www.rethink.org/living_with_mental_illness/everyday_living/stigma_mental_illness/stigma_and_1.html

Rice V.H. & Stead L.F. (2008). Nursing interventions for smoking cessation. Cochrane Database of Systematic Reviews 2008, Issue 1. Art. No.: CD001188. DOI: 10.1002/14651858. CD001188.pub3.

Rigotti N.A., Munafo M.R. & Stead L.F. (2007). Interventions for smoking cessation in hospitalised patients. Cochrane Database of Systematic Reviews 2007, Issue 3. Art. No.: CD001837.DOI:10.1002/14651837.pub2.

Rihs M., Muller C. & Baumann P. (1996). Caffeine consumption in hospitalised psychiatric patients. European Arch Psychiatry Clinical Neurosciences 246, 83–92.

Ritchie J., Dick D. & Lingham R. (1994). The report of the inquiry into the care and treatment of Christopher clunis. HMSO, London.

Rogers A. & Pilgrim D. (1994) Service users' views of psychiatric nurses. British Journal of Nursing 3(1), 16–18.

Rollnick S., Mason P. & Butler C. (2000). Health Behaviour Change: A Guide for Practitioners. Churchill Livingstone, Edinburgh.

Rose D. (2001). Users' Voices: The Perspectives of Mental Health Service Users on Community and Hospital Care. SCMH, London.

Royal College of Nursing (2007). A Joint statement on continuing professional development (CPD) for health and social care practitioners. RCN, London.

Royal College of Psychiatrists (2002). Annual census of psychiatric staffing 2001. Occasional paper 54. RCP, London.

Royal College of Psychiatrists (2007). Accreditation for Acute Inpatients Mental Health Services (AIMS). Accessed at: http://www.rcpsych.ac.uk/AIMS

Running A., Kipp C. & Mercer V. (2006). Prescriptive patterns of nurse practitioners and physicians. Journal of the American Academy of Nurse Practitioners 18, 228–233.

Rutter M. & Quinton D. (1984). Parental psychiatric disorder: effects on children. Psychological Medicine 14, 853–880.

Ryan A.A. & Chambers M. (2000). Medication management and older patients: an individualised and systematic approach. Journal of Clinical Nursing 9, 732–741.

Ryan M.C.M. & Thakore J.H. (2002). Physical consequences of schizophrenia and its treatment. The metabolic syndrome. Life Sciences 71, 239–257.

Ryan-Woolley B., McHugh G. & Luker K.A. (2007). Prescribing by specialist nurses in cancer and palliative care: results of a national survey. Palliative Medicine 21, 273–277.

Saari K., Koponen H., Laitinen J., et al. (2004). Hyperlipidaemia in persons using antipsychotic medication: a general population-based birth cohort study. Journal of Clinical Psychiatry 65, 547–550.

Sainsbury Centre for Mental Health (2001). The capable practitioner. SCMH, London.

Sainsbury Centre for Mental Health (2003). The search for acute solutions: a project to improve and evaluate acute mental health inpatient care. SCMH, London.

Sainsbury Centre for Mental Health (2005). Acute care: a national survey of adult psychiatric wards in England. SCMH, London.

Saitz R., Palfai T.N.F., Winter M.R., et al. (2007). Screening and brief interventions online for college students: the health study. Alcohol 42, 28–36.

Samson C. (1995). The fracturing of medical dominance in British psychiatry. Sociology of Health & Illness 17, 245–268.

Sawynok J. (1995). Pharmacological rationale for the clinical use of caffeine. Drugs 49, 37–50.

Schmidt I., Claesson C.B., Westerholm B., et al. (1998). The impact of regular multidisciplinary team interventions on psychotropic drugs in Swedish nursing homes. Journal of American Geriatric Society 46, 77–82.

Schou M. (1997). Forty years of lithium treatment. Archives of General Psychiatry 54, 9–13.

Scott J., Teasdale J.D., Paykel E.S., et al. (2000). Effects of cognitive therapy on psychological symptoms and social functioning in residual symptoms. British Journal of Psychiatry 177, 440–446.

Scull A.T. (1979). Museums of Madness: The Social Organization of Insanity in Nineteenth-century England. Allen Lane.

Sernyak M., Leslie D., Alarcan R., et al. (2002). Association of diabetes mellitus with use of atypical neuroleptics in the treatment of schizophrenia. American Journal of Psychiatry 159, 561–566.

Shoptaw S., Rotheram-Fuller E., Yang X., et al. (2002). Smoking cessation in methadone maintenance. Addiction 97, 1317–1328.

Silverman K., Evans S.M., Strain E.C., et al. (1992). Withdrawal syndrome after the double-blind cessation of caffeine consumption. The New England Journal of Medicine 327, 1109–1114.

Silverstone T., Smith G. & Goodall E. (1988). Prevalence of obesity in patients receiving depot antipsychotics. British Journal of Psychiatry 153, 214–217.

Simpson G.M. & Angus J.W. (1970). A rating scale for extrapyramidal side effects. Acta Psychiatrica Scandinavica 212, 11–19.

Siriwardena A.N. (2006). The rise and rise of non-medical prescribing. Quality in Primary Care 14(1), 1–3.

Skingsley D., Bradley E. & Nolan P. (2006). Neuropharmacology and mental health nurse prescribers. Journal of Clinical Nursing 15(8), 989–997.

Snowden A. (2007). Why mental health nurses should prescribe. Nurse Prescribing 5, 193–198.

Sodha M., McLaughlin M., Williams G., et al. (2002). Nurses' confidence and pharmacological knowledge: a study. British Journal of Community Nursing 7, 309–315.

Solomon D.A., Keller M.B. & Leon A.C. (2000). Multiple recurrence of major depressive disorder. American Journal of Psychiatry 157, 229–233.

Stahl S.M. (2000). Essential Psychopharmacology: Neuroscientific Basis and Practical Applications, 2nd edition. Cambridge University Press, Cambridge.

Stahl S.M. (2003). Primary care companion. Journal of Clinical Psychiatry 5(Suppl 3), 9–13.

Stahl S.M. (2006). Essential Psychopharmacology: The Prescribers Guide. Cambridge University Press, Cambridge.

Standing Nursing and Midwifery Advisory Committee (SNMAC) (1999). Mental health nursing: Addressing acute concerns. Report by the Standing Nursing and Midwifery Advisory Committee. Department of Health, London.

Stenner K. & Courntenay M. (2008). Benefits of nurse prescribing for patients in pain: nurses' views. Journal of Advanced Nursing 63, 27–35.

Sussman N. (2001). Review of atypical antipsychotics and weight gain. Journal of Clinical Psychiatry 62, 5–12.

Talley S. & Brooke P.S. (1992). Prescriptive authority for psychiatric clinical specialists: framing the issues. Archives of Psychiatric Nursing VI(2), 71–82.

Talley S. & Richens S. (2001). Prescribing practices of advanced practice psychiatric nurses: part 1 – demographic, educational and practice characteristics. Archives of Psychiatric Nursing XV(5), 205–213.

Tamminga C.A. & Lahti A.C. (1996). The new generation of antipsychotic drugs. International Clinical Psychopharmacology 11, 73–76.

Tanskanen A., Hibbeln J.R., Hintikka J., et al. (2001). Fish consumption, depression and suicidality in a general population. Archives of General Psychiatry 58, 512–513.

Taylor D., Paton C. & Kerwin R. (2007). Prescribing Guidelines, 9th edition. Taylor & Francis, London.

Thornicroft G. (2006). Perceptions by service users of healthcare staff. Accessed at: http://www.mentalhealthcare.org.uk/content/?id=191

Thornley B. & Adams C. (1998). Content and quality of 2000 controlled trials in schizophrenia over 50 years. British Medical Journal 317, 1181–1184.

Toma R., Jakovljevic T. & Brimblecombe N. (2008). Psychiatrists' and nurses' views of mental health nurse supplementary prescribing: a survey. Psychiatric Bulletin 32, 364–365.

Tompkins M. (2004). Using homework in psychotherapy: Strategies, Guidelines and Forms. The Guildford Press, London.

Tonna A.P., Steward D., West B., et al. (2007). Pharmacist prescribing in the UK – a literature review of current practice and research. Journal of Clinical Pharmacy and Therapeutics 32, 545–556.

Turner B.S. (1987). Medical power and social knowledge. Sage, London.

Turner D. (2002). Mapping the routes to recovery. Mental Health Today July, 29–30.

Tyrer P. & Steinberg D. (2005). Models for mental disorder. John Wiley & Sons, Chichester.

Usher K., Foster K. & McNamara P. (2005). Antipsychotic drugs and pregnant or breastfeeding women: issues for mental health nurses. Journal of Psychiatric and Mental Health Nursing 12, 713–718.

Ustun T.B., Ayuso-Matoes J.L., Chatterji S., et al. (2000). Global burden of depressive disorders in the year 2000. British Journal of Psychiatry 184, 386–392.

Ustun T.B. and Chatterji S. (2001). Global burden of depressive disorders and future projections. In: A. Dawson & A. Tylee (Eds.). Depression: Social and Economic Time Bomb. BMJ Books, London.

Venning P., Durie A., Roland M. et al. (2000). Randomised controlled trial comparing cost effectiveness of general practitioners and nurse practitioners in primary care. British Medical Journal 320, 1048–1053.

Vincent C., Neale G. & Woloshynowych M. (2001). Adverse events in British hospitals: preliminary retrospective review. British Medical Journal 322, 517–519.

Walburn J., Gray R., Gournay K., et al. (2001). Systematic review of patient and nurse attitudes to depot antipsychotic medication. British Journal of Psychiatry 179, 300–307.

Wand T. & White K. (2007). Progression of the mental health nurse practitioner role in Australia. Journal of Psychiatric and Mental Health Nursing 14, 644–651.

Wanless D. (2002). Securing Our Future Health: Taking a Long-Term View. Her Majesty's Treasury, London.

Welch R. & Chue P. (2000). Antipsychotic agents and QT changes. Journal of Psychiatry Neurosciences 25, 154–160.

Wells J., Gooney M., Bergen J., et al. (In press). Views on nurse prescribing – a report of a survey of community mental health nurses in the Republic of Ireland. Journal of Psychiatric and Mental Health Nursing.

While A.E. & Biggs K.S.M. (2004). Benefits and challenges of nurse prescribing. Journal of Advanced Nursing 45, 559–567.

Whiting J. (2007). Nursing the homeless: health care on the streets. Nurse Prescribing 11, 485–487.

Wieck A. & Haddad P.M. (2003). Antipsychotic-induced hyperprolactinaemia in women: pathophysiology, severity and consequences. British Journal of Psychiatry 182, 199–204.

Wilhelmsson S. & Foldevi M. (2003). Exploring views on Swedish district nurses' prescribing – a focus group study in primary health care. Journal of Clinical Nursing 12(5), 643–650.

Wilkinson G., Moore B. & Moore P. (1990). Treating People with Depression: A Practical Guide for Primary Care. Radcliffe Medical Press, Oxon.

Wilson J. (1996). A look up the scope. Nursing Management 2(8), 16–17.

Wing J.K., Cooper J.E. & Sartorius N. (1974). Measurement and Classification of Psychiatric Symptoms: An Instruction Manual for the PSE and the CATEGO Programme. Cambridge University Press, London.

Wirshing D.A., Pierre J.M., Erhart S.M., et al. (2003). Understanding the new and evolving profile of adverse drug effects in schizophrenia. Psychiatric Clinics of North America 26, 165–190.

Wittchen H.U. & Jacobi F. (2005). Size and burden of mental disorders in Europe: a critical review and appraisal of 27 studies. Neuropsychopharmacology 15, 357–376.

Wix S. (2007). Independent nurse prescribing in the mental health setting. Nursing Times 103, 30–31.

Wong F. & Chung L. (2006). Establishing a definition for a nurse-led clinic: structure, process, and outcome. Journal of Advanced Nursing 53, 358–369.

World Cancer Research Fund (2007). Food, nutrition, physical activity and the prevention of cancer: a global perspective. WCRF, London.

World Health Organisation (2001). Mental health: new understanding, new hope. World Health Organisation, Geneva.

World Health Organisation (2002). Reducing risks, promoting healthy life. World Health Organisation, Geneva.

World Health Organisation (2007). BMI classification. World Health Organisation, Geneva.

Wu M.-K., Wang C.-K., Bai Y.-C., et al. (2007). Outcomes of obese, clozapine-treated inpatients with schizophrenia placed on a six-month diet and physical activity program. Psychiatric Services 58, 544–551.

Young R.C., Biggs J.T., Ziegler V.E., et al. (1978). A rating scale for mania: reliability, validity and sensitivity. British Journal of Psychiatry 133, 429–435.

Young Y. (2005). Lipids for psychiatrists – an overview. Journal of Psychopharmacology 19, 66–75.

Zimmet P., Alberti G. & Shaw J. (2005). A new IDF worldwide definition of the metabolic syndrome: the rationale and the results. Diabetes Voice 50, 31–33.

Zubin J. & Spring B. (1977). Vulnerability – a new view of schizophrenia. Journal of Abnormal Psychology 86, 103–124.

Zucconi M. & Ferini-Strambi L. (2004). Epidemiology and clinical findings of restless leg syndrome. Sleep Medicine 5(3), 293–299.

Zwarenstein M. & Reeves S. (2006). Knowledge translation and interprofessional collaboration: where the rubber of evidence-based care hits the road of teamwork. Journal of Continuing Education in the Health Professions 26, 46–54.

Index